This book is dedicated to

President Dwight D. Eisenhower

for reasons set forth in chapter 1.

PENGUIN BOOKS

THE HEALING OF AMERICA

T. R. Reid is a longtime correspondent for *The Washington Post* and former chief of its Tokyo and London bureaus, as well as a commentator for National Public Radio. His books include *The United States of Europe*, *The Chip*, and *Confucius Lives Next Door*.

Praise for *The Healing of America*

"*The Healing of America* cuts, with the skill of a brilliant surgeon, through the myths and misunderstandings surrounding the American health-care crisis. . . . This is a book that everyone should read before taking sides in the debate about an issue that, for many of us, is nothing less than a matter of life and death."

—Francine Prose, *O, The Oprah Magazine*

"This book's clarity, comprehensiveness, and readability are exceptional, and its bottom line is a little different from most. Instead of rationalization and hand-wringing, Mr. Reid offers an array of possible solutions for our crisis. As the proverb goes (it is a favorite among policy wonks): 'To find your way in the fog, follow the tracks of the oxcart ahead.' We have plenty of reasonable paths to follow."

—Abigail Zuger, M.D., *The New York Times*

"An extremely good, and extremely readable, explanation of how our system compares to those of other countries."   —*The Washington Post*

"*The Healing of America* could have been a policy-heavy slog, but Reid manages to keep it low on wonkery, crisply paced, and seriously incisive. Reid's book couldn't be more timely." —*Business Week*

"[*The Healing of America*] makes a critically important contribution to the conversation about reform by taking a clear-eyed look at what is actually working in other countries." —*The Christian Science Monitor*

"I would urge Penguin Press to sprinkle advance copies liberally throughout Congress, the White House, and the Health and Human Services department." —*Slate*

"It's the clearest and most useful contribution to the ongoing health-care reform debate that I've read. And, unlike most books that are described as a 'useful contribution,' it's a good read, too." —Ezra Klein, *B&N Review*

"Reid writes engagingly and lightens his text by recounting his visits to doctors in different countries for help with his bum shoulder." —Bloomberg.com

"Whether you're primed to agree with Reid's bleak assessment of the U.S. health-care system or not, his perspective—both global and intimate—makes for worthwhile and timely reading." —*Los Angeles Times*

"Reid dispels the common fears about 'socialized medicine,' waiting lists, and other myths disseminated by the lobbyists and politicians with a stake in the status quo. Here, we get a clear picture of why we have a moral imperative to implement a health-care system for all Americans." —*Booklist*

"A reasoned, well-balanced, highly readable account, especially welcome as the national debate over health care gets underway." —*Kirkus Reviews* (starred review)

THE HEALING
OF AMERICA

A GLOBAL QUEST
FOR BETTER, CHEAPER,
AND FAIRER HEALTH CARE

T. R. Reid

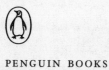

PENGUIN BOOKS

PENGUIN BOOKS

Published by the Penguin Group

Penguin Group (USA) Inc., 375 Hudson Street, New York, New York 10014, U.S.A.

Penguin Group (Canada), 90 Eglinton Avenue East, Suite 700, Toronto,
Ontario, Canada M4P 2Y3 (a division of Pearson Penguin Canada Inc.)

Penguin Books Ltd, 80 Strand, London WC2R 0RL, England

Penguin Ireland, 25 St Stephen's Green, Dublin 2, Ireland (a division of Penguin Books Ltd)

Penguin Group (Australia), 250 Camberwell Road, Camberwell,
Victoria 3124, Australia (a division of Pearson Australia Group Pty Ltd)

Penguin Books India Pvt Ltd, 11 Community Centre, Panchsheel Park, New Delhi – 110 017, India

Penguin Group (NZ), 67 Apollo Drive, Rosedale, North Shore 0632,
New Zealand (a division of Pearson New Zealand Ltd)

Penguin Books (South Africa) (Pty) Ltd, 24 Sturdee Avenue,
Rosebank, Johannesburg 2196, South Africa

Penguin Books Ltd, Registered Offices:
80 Strand, London WC2R 0RL, England

First published in the United States of America by The Penguin Press,
a member of Penguin Group (USA) Inc. 2009
This edition with a new afterword published in Penguin Books 2010

10 9 8 7 6

THE LIBRARY OF CONGRESS HAS CATALOGED THE HARDCOVER EDITION AS FOLLOWS:
Reid, T. R.
The healing of America : a global quest for better, cheaper, and fairer health care / T. R. Reid
p.   cm.
Includes bibliographical references and index.
ISBN 978-1-59420-234-6 (hc.)
ISBN 978-0-14-311821-3 (pbk.)
1. Medical policy—United States.   2. Health care reform—United States.
3. Medical care—United States.   I. Title.
[DNLM: 1. Delivery of Health Care—United States.   2. Developed Countries—United States.
3. Health Care Reform—United States.   4. Universal Coverage—United States.
W   84.1   R358h   2009]
RA395.A3R435 2009   2009009555
362.10973—dc22

Printed in the United States of America
Designed by Meighan Cavanaugh

Contents

THE HEALING OF AMERICA

Prologue:
A Moral Question

IF NIKKI WHITE HAD BEEN A RESIDENT OF ANY OTHER rich country, she would be alive today.

Around the time she graduated from college, Monique A. "Nikki" White contracted systemic lupus erythematosus; that's a serious disease, but one that modern medicine knows how to manage. If this bright, feisty, dazzling young woman had lived in, say, Japan—the world's second-richest nation—or Germany (third richest), or Britain, France, Italy, Spain, Canada, Sweden, etc., the health care systems there would have given her the standard treatment for lupus, and she could have lived a normal life span. But Nikki White was a citizen of the world's richest country, the United States of America. Once she was sick, she couldn't get health insurance. Like tens of millions of her fellow Americans, she had too much money to qualify for health care under welfare, but too little money to pay for the drugs and doctors she needed to stay alive. She spent the last months of her life frantically writing letters and filling out forms, pleading for help. When she died, Nikki White was thirty-two years old.

"Nikki didn't die from lupus," Dr. Amylyn Crawford told me. "It was a lack of access to health care that killed Nikki White." Dr. Crawford is a family physician at a no-frills community health center in an old strip mall in a downscale section of Kingsport, Tennessee. She sees lots of hard cases. Still, she couldn't stop sobbing as she recalled her late patient Monique White: "I told Nikki that she had lupus. But I also told her that a diagnosis of lupus is not a death sentence. If Nikki had not lost her health insurance, she'd be alive today."

Later in this book, we'll take a detailed look at Nikki White's tragic encounter with America's health care system. But the larger tragedy is that Ms. White is not alone. Government and academic studies report that more than twenty thousand Americans die in the prime of life each year from medical problems that could be treated, because they can't afford to see a doctor. On September 11, 2001, some three thousand Americans were killed by terrorists; our country has spent hundreds of billions of dollars to make sure it doesn't happen again. But that same year, and every year since then, some twenty thousand Americans died because they couldn't get health care. That doesn't happen in any other developed country. Hundreds of thousands of Americans go bankrupt every year because of medical bills. That doesn't happen in any other developed country either.

Those Americans who die or go broke because they happened to get sick represent a fundamental moral decision our country has made. Despite all the rights and privileges and entitlements that Americans enjoy today, we have never decided to provide medical care for everybody who needs it. The far-reaching health care reform that Congress passed in 2010 is designed to increase coverage substantially—but it will still leave about 23 million Americans uninsured. Even when "Obamacare" takes full effect, the American health care system will still lead to large numbers of avoidable deaths and bankruptcies among our fellow citizens. As we saw in the national debate over that bill, efforts to increase coverage tend to be derailed by arguments about "big government" or "free enterprise" or "socialism"—and the essential moral question gets lost in the shouting.

All the other developed countries on earth have made a different moral decision. All the other countries like us—that is, wealthy, technologically advanced, industrialized democracies—guarantee medical care to anyone who gets sick. Countries that are just as committed as we are to equal opportunity, individual liberty, and the free market have concluded that everybody has a right to health care—and they provide it. One result is that most rich countries have better national health statistics—longer life expectancy, lower infant mortality, better recovery rates from major diseases—than the United States does. Yet all the other rich countries spend far less on health care than the United States does.

Contrary to conventional American wisdom, most developed countries manage health care without resorting to "socialized medicine." How do they do it? That's what this book is about. I set out on a global tour of doctors' offices and hospitals and health ministries to see how the other industrialized democracies organize health care systems that are universal, affordable, and effective.

My global quest made it clear that the other wealthy democracies can show us how to build a decent health care system—if that's what we want. The design of any nation's health care system involves political, economic, and medical decisions. But the primary issue for any health care system is a moral one. If we want to fix American health care, we first have to answer a basic question: Should we guarantee medical treatment to everyone who needs it? Or should we let Americans like Nikki White die from "a lack of access to health care"? Once we settle that point, the nations we'll visit in this book can show us how to manage the mechanics of universal health care. We don't need a carbon copy of any particular country's health care system; rather, we can draw valuable lessons from each of the models described in this book. If Americans can find the political will to provide health care for everybody, the rest of the world can show us the way.

ONE

A Quest for Two Cures

MRS. RAMA CAME SWEEPING INTO MY HOSPITAL ROOM with the haughty grandeur of a Brahmin empress, wearing a salmon pink sari and leading a retinue of assistants, interpreters, and equipment bearers. It wasn't exactly medical equipment they were carrying, because Mrs. Rama wasn't exactly a doctor. Still, her professional services were considered an essential element of the medical regimen at India's famous Arya Vaidya Chikitsalayam, the Mayo Clinic of traditional Indian medicine. Indeed, Mrs. Rama's diagnostic work is covered by Indian medical insurance. As she set up her equipment—on a painted wooden board, she carefully arranged a collection of shells, rocks, and statuettes of Hindu gods—Mrs. Rama told me that she was connected to the clinic's Department of Yajnopathy, an ancient Indian specialty that roughly equates to astrology. Her medical role was to ascertain my place in the cosmos; in that way, she could determine whether the timing was propitious for me to be healed. Any fool could see, she explained in matter-of-fact tones, that it would be a mistake to proceed with medical treatment if the stars in heaven were aligned against me.

For all her majestic self-assurance, Mrs. Rama did not immediately inspire confidence in her patient. After asking some basic questions, she shuffled the stones and statuettes around her checkerboard and launched into my diagnosis. "In the summer of 1986, you got married," she declared firmly. Well, not exactly. In the summer of 1986, my wife and I celebrated our fourteenth wedding anniversary; by then we had three kids, a dog, and a minivan. "In 1998," she went on, "you were far from home and were treated for serious illness." Well, not exactly. Our American family was, in fact, living in London in 1998; but in that whole year, I never saw a doctor.

Mrs. Rama kept talking, but I stopped listening. To me, the stones and shells and statues all seemed preposterous. Still, I kept my mouth shut. If Indian medicine required yajnopathic analysis before health care could begin (and Mrs. Rama did eventually conclude that the timing was propitious for treatment), that was fine with me. I was willing to go along, in pursuit of the greater goal. For I had traveled to the Arya Vaidya clinic—it's in the state of Tamil Nadu, at the southern tip of the subcontinent, where the Bay of Bengal meets the Arabian Sea—on a kind of medical pilgrimage. I was on a global quest, searching for solutions to two different health problems, one personal and one of national dimensions.

On the personal level, I was hoping to find some relief for my ailing right shoulder, which I bashed badly decades ago as a seaman, second class, in the U.S. Navy. In 1972, a navy surgeon (literally) screwed the joint back together, and that repair job worked fine for a while. Over time, though, the stainless-steel screw in my clavicle loosened; my shoulder grew increasingly painful and hard to move. By the first decade of the twenty-first century, I could no longer swing a golf club. I could barely reach up to replace a lightbulb overhead or get the wineglasses from the top shelf. Yearning for surcease from sorrow, I took that bum shoulder to doctors and clinics—including Mrs. Rama's *chikitsalayam*—in countries around the world.

The quest began at home. I went to a brilliant American orthopedist, Dr. Donald Ferlic, a specialist who had skillfully repaired another broken joint of mine a few years back. Dr. Ferlic proposed a surgical intervention that reflects precisely the high-tech ethos of contemporary American medicine. This operation—it is known as a total shoulder arthroplasty, Procedure No. 080.81 on the National Center for Health Statistics' roster of "clinical modifications"—would require the orthopedist to take a surgical saw, cut off the shoulder joint that God gave me, and replace it with a man-made contraption of silicon and titanium. This new arthroplastic joint would be hammered into my upper arm and then cemented to my clavicle. The doctor was confident that this would reduce my shoulder pain—orthopedic surgeons tend to be confident by nature—but I had serious reservations about Procedure No. 080.81. The saws and hammers and glue made the operation sound rather drastic. It would cost tens of thousands of dollars (like most major medical procedures in the United States, the exact price was veiled in mystery). The best prognosis I could get was that the operation might or might not give me more shoulder movement. And when I asked Dr. Ferlic what could go wrong in the course of a total arthroplasty, he was completely honest. "Well, you have all the risks that go with major surgery," he answered frankly. And then he listed the risks: Disease. Paralysis. Death.

With that, a certain skepticism crept into my soul about this high-tech medical intervention. I departed my American surgeon's office and took my aching shoulder to other doctors, doctors all over the globe. Over the next year or so, I had my blood pressure and temperature taken in ten different languages. I ran into a world of different diagnostic techniques, ranging from Mrs. Rama and her star charts to a diligent, studious doctor (we'll meet him in chapter 9) who told me he couldn't possibly analyze my medical condition without tasting my urine. In Taipei, an acupuncturist twirled her needles in my left knee to treat the pain in my right shoulder. The shoulder itself was examined, X-rayed, patted, poked, palpated, massaged, and manipulated in countless ways. Some of these treatments worked, more or less; as we'll see in chapter 9, Mrs. Rama's colleagues at the *chikitsalayam* were helpful. Others proved no help at all.

THIS WAS NOT A major disappointment, though, because that aching shoulder was really just a secondary impetus for my medical odyssey. It would be ridiculous, after all, to go all the way to the southern tip of India—not to mention London, Paris, Berlin, Tokyo, and so on—to get treatment for a sore shoulder that isn't, frankly, all that sore. The stiffness is tolerable most of the time. I have another arm to use for changing lightbulbs or getting glasses off the shelf. I don't have a golf swing anymore, but even when I could swing a club I was a rotten golfer.

So the shoulder was not my top priority. Rather, the primary goal of my travels was to find a solution to a much bigger medical problem. It's a national problem—a national scandal, really—that is undermining the physical and fiscal health of every American. With help from many scholars and the Kaiser Family Foundation, I traveled the world searching for a prescription to fix our country's seriously ailing health care system. As Nikki White's experience demonstrates, it's fundamentally a moral problem: We've created a health care system that leaves millions of our fellow citizens out in the cold. Beyond the issue of coverage, however, the United States also performs below other wealthy countries in matters of cost, quality, and choice.

Most Americans can remember when our politicians used to boast—and we used to believe—that the United States had "the finest health care system in the world." Today, any U.S. politician who dared to make that claim—it was last heard in a State of the Union address in 2002—would be hooted out of the room. Americans generally recognize now that our nation's health care system has become excessively expensive, ineffective, and unjust. Among the world's developed nations, the United States stands at or near the bottom in most important rankings of access to and quality of medical care. In 2000, when a Harvard Medical School professor working at the World Health Organization developed a complicated formula to rate the quality and fairness of national health care systems around the world, the richest nation on earth ranked thirty-seventh.[1] That placed us just behind Dominica and Costa Rica, and just ahead of Slovenia and Cuba. France came in first. (For more about the WHO's global ranking, see the appendix.)

The one area where the United States unquestionably leads the world is in spending. Even countries with considerably older populations than ours, with more need for medical attention, spend much less than we do. Japan has the oldest population in the world, and the Japanese go to the doctor more than anybody—about fourteen office

HEALTH EXPENDITURE AS A PERCENTAGE OF GDP, 2005

USA	16.5
France	11.0
Switzerland	10.8
Germany	10.4
Canada	10.1
Sweden	9.1
UK	8.4
Japan	8.1
Mexico	7.3
Taiwan	6.2

Sources: OECD Health at a Glance, 2009; Government of Taiwan.

visits per year, compared with five for the average American. And yet Japan spends about $3,400 per person on health care each year; we burn through $7,400 per person.

There's nothing particularly wrong with spending a lot of money on something important, as long as you get a decent return for what you spend. It's certainly not wasteful to spend money for effective medical treatment. If a dentist who was about to drill a tooth offered her patient a choice between listening to pleasant music for free to lessen the pain, or a shot of Novocain for $50, most people would pay for the shot and would probably get their money's worth. And there's nothing wrong with paying more for better performance. Those fifty-two-inch high-definition plasma televisions that people hang on the family room wall these days cost five times what a top-of-the-line set would have cost ten years ago, but buyers are willing to shell out the extra money because the enhanced viewing quality is worth the price.

When it comes to medical care, though, Americans are shelling out the big bucks without getting what we pay for. As we'll see shortly, the quality of medical care that Americans buy is often inferior to the treatment people get in other countries. And patients know it. Surveys show that Americans who see a doctor tend to be less satisfied with their treatment than Britons, Italians, Germans, Canadians, or the Japanese—even though we pay the doctor much more than they do.[2]

When Barack Obama entered the White House in January of 2009, it seemed as if the stars were aligned and the timing was propitious for the United States to establish a new national health care system. Obama had made health care reform a central pillar of his presidential campaign, and exit polls on election day in 2008 showed that nearly 80 percent of voters wanted substantial changes in the U.S. medical system.[3] In fact, though, the new president's health care proposals prompted ferocious national debate and finally squeaked through Congress without a single vote to spare. So many compromises had to be made along the way to passage that the new bill still falls short of universal coverage.

The thesis of this book is that we can find cost-effective ways to cover every American by borrowing ideas from foreign models of health care. For me, that conclusion stems from personal experience. I've worked overseas for years as a foreign correspondent; our family has lived on three continents, and we've used the health care systems in other wealthy countries with satisfaction. But many Americans intensely dislike the idea that we might learn useful policy ideas from other countries, particularly in medicine. The leaders of the health care industry and the medical profession, not to mention the political establishment, have a single, all-purpose response they fall back on whenever somebody suggests that the United States might usefully study foreign health care systems: "But it's socialized medicine!"[4]

This is supposed to end the argument. The contention is that the United States, with its commitment to free markets and low taxes, could never rely on big-government socialism the way other countries do. Americans have learned in school that the private sector can handle things better and more efficiently than government ever could. In U.S. policy debates, the term "socialized medicine" has been a powerful political weapon—even though nobody can quite define what it means. The term was popularized by a public relations firm working for the American Medical Association in 1947 to disparage President Truman's proposal for a national health care system. It was a label, at the dawn of the cold war, meant to suggest that anybody advocating universal access to health care must be a communist. And the phrase has retained its political power for six decades.

There are two basic flaws, though, in this argument.

1. Most national health care systems are not "socialized." As we'll see, many foreign countries provide universal health care of high quality at reasonable cost using private doctors, private hospitals, and private insurance plans. Some countries offering universal coverage have a smaller government role than the

United States does. Americans switch to government-run Medicare when they turn sixty-five; in Germany and Switzerland, seniors stick with their private insurers no matter how old they are. Even where government plays a large role, doctors' offices are operated as private businesses. As we'll see in chapter 7, my doctor in London, Dr. Ahmed Badat, was nobody's socialist; he was a fiercely entrepreneurial capitalist who regularly found ways to enhance his income within the National Health Service. Many countries have privately owned hospitals, some run by charities, some for profit; Japan has more for-profit hospitals than the United States.

In short, the universal health care systems in developed countries around the world are not nearly as "socialized" as the health insurance industry and the American Medical Association want you to think.

2. "Socialized medicine" may be a scary term, but in practice, Americans rather like government-run medicine. The U.S. Department of Veterans Affairs is one of the world's purest models of socialized medicine at work. In the Medicare system, covering about 44 million elderly or disabled Americans, the federal government makes the rules and pays the bills. And yet both of these "socialized" health care systems are enormously popular with the people who use them and consistently rate high in surveys of patient satisfaction. During the debate over "Obamacare," even those who complained most angrily about a "government takeover of health care" insisted that Medicare and the VA must continue to be government-run systems.

So the problem isn't "socialism." The real problem with those foreign health care systems is that they're foreign. That offends the mind-set—sometimes referred to as American exceptionalism—that says our strong, wealthy, and enormously productive country is sui generis and doesn't need to borrow any ideas from the rest of the world. Anybody who dares to say that other countries do something better than we do is likely to be labeled unpatriotic or anti-American; I've run into that charge myself. Of course, this is nonsense. The real patriot, the person who genuinely loves his country, or college, or company, is the person who recognizes its problems and tries to fix them. Often, the best way to solve a problem is to study what other colleges, companies, or countries have done. And the fact is, Americans often do look overseas for good ideas. We have borrowed numerous foreign innovations that have become staples of American daily life: public broadcasting, text messaging, pizza, sushi, yoga, reality TV, *The Office,* and even *American Idol.*

The academics have a term for this approach to problem-solving: "comparative policy analysis." The patron saint of comparative policy analysis was an American military hero who went on to become our thirty-fourth president: Dwight D. Eisenhower. That's why this book is dedicated to his memory.

When Eisenhower became president, in 1953, the key domestic issue was the sorry state of the nation's transit infrastructure. Almost all major highways then were two-lane country roads designed primarily to get farmers' crops to the nearest market. Interstate travel was a torturous ordeal, marked by rickety bridges and long stretches of mud or gravel between intermittent paved sections. As postwar America embraced the automobile, it was clear that vast improvements were required. And most of the forty-eight states already had highway plans on the books. For the most part, those blueprints called for networks of two-lane highways that would run through the downtown Main Street of every city along the route. These were perfectly reasonable plans for the time. But Eisenhower, who recognized the value of comparative policy analysis, had a better idea.

As Supreme Allied Commander during World War II, Ike had commanded the long push by American and British soldiers toward

Berlin after the D-day landings in June 1944. By the spring of 1945, the Allies had battled their way across France to Germany's western border. Eisenhower's strategic plan envisioned months of painful slogging across a shattered German countryside. But then his forward commanders reported an amazing discovery: a broad ribbon of highway, the best road system anybody had ever seen, stretching straight through the heart of Germany. This was the autobahn network, built in the 1930s, which featured four-lane highways; overpasses and ramped interchanges to avoid intersections; and rest areas for refueling every hundred miles or so. Once Eisenhower's trucks, tanks, and troop carriers found the superhighway, they moved much faster than Ike had planned. By early May of 1945, the war in Europe was over.

Those German roads came to mind when, in 1953, President Eisenhower was presented with rather timid plans for a two-lane highway network across America. "After seeing the autobahns of modern Germany, and knowing the assets those highways were to the Germans," he wrote in his memoirs, "I decided, as President, to put an emphasis on this kind of road-building. I made a personal and absolute decision to see that the nation would benefit from it. The [American plans] had started me thinking about good, two-lane highways, but Germany had made me see the wisdom of broader ribbons across the land."[5] So Eisenhower built those "broader ribbons": a state-of-the-art network designed to a single national standard, with four-lane divided highways; overpasses and ramped interchanges to avoid intersections; and rest areas for refueling every hundred miles or so. There was considerable debate about how to pay for this hugely ambitious engineering project. A giant bond issue was proposed. But in those more innocent times, it was considered irresponsible for the federal government to run up large debts; in the end, Ike settled on a highway trust fund financed by gasoline taxes.

Today, the interstates—formally designated the Dwight D. Eisenhower System of Interstate and Defense Highways—comprise 47,000 miles of road, 55,500 bridges, 14,750 interchanges, and zero stop-lights. The system has spawned such basic elements of American life as the suburb, the motel, the chain store, the recreational vehicle, the automotive seat belt, the spring-break trek to Florida, the thirty-mile commute to work, and, on the dark side, the two-mile-long traf-fic jam. It's one of the finest highway networks in the world—and nobody seems to care that the basic idea was copied from the Nazis.[6]

EISENHOWER, THE PRAGMATIC COMMANDER, was willing to borrow a good policy idea, even if it had foreign lineage. In the same spirit, my sore shoulder and I hit the road, looking for good ideas for managing a nation's health care. But where should I look?

TWO

Different Models, Common Principles

EACH NATION'S HEALTH CARE SYSTEM IS A REFLECTION OF its history, politics, economy, and national values. Canada's universal program is notorious for keeping patients on waiting lists; but Canadians, with their egalitarian traditions, have decided they would rather keep patients waiting in line—as long as everybody waits about the same amount of time—than see some people get treatment immediately and some not at all. The British are adamant that nobody should have to pay a medical bill. The UK's National Health Service has always held true to its founding principle: "Free at the point of service." But just twenty-five miles across the Channel, the French are equally adamant that people should pay some fee for virtually every medical service, even though that fee will be reimbursed in whole or part in a matter of days by the insurance system. British women tend to have their babies at home; Japanese women, in contrast, almost always give birth in the hospital—and mother and child remain there for five to ten days after delivery.

Fortunately, for all the local variations, health care systems tend to follow general patterns. In some models, government is both the provider of health care and the payer. In others, doctors and hospitals are in the private sector but government pays the bills. In still other countries, both the providers and the payers are private. There are four basic arrangements:

THE BISMARCK MODEL

This system—found in Germany, Japan, Belgium, Switzerland, and, to a degree, in Latin America—is named for the Prussian chancellor Otto von Bismarck, who invented the welfare state as part of the unification of Germany in the nineteenth century. Despite its European heritage, the model would look familiar to Americans. In Bismarck countries, both health care providers and payers are private entitites. The model uses private health insurance plans, usually financed jointly by employers and employees through payroll deduction. Unlike the U.S. health insurance industry, though, Bismarck-type plans are basically charities: They cover everybody, and they don't make a profit. The doctor's office is a private business, and many hospitals are privately owned. Although this is a multipayer model (Germany has more than two hundred funds), tight regulation of medical services and fees gives the system much of the cost-control clout that the single-payer Beveridge Model (see below) provides.

THE BEVERIDGE MODEL

This arrangement is named after William Beveridge, a daring social reformer (we'll meet him in chapter 7) who inspired Britain's National Health Service. In this system, health care is provided and financed by the government, through tax payments. There are no medical bills;

rather, medical treatment is a public service, like the fire department or the public library. In Beveridge systems, many (sometimes all) hospitals and clinics are owned by the government; some doctors are government employees, but there are also private doctors who collect their fees from the government. These systems tend to have low costs per capita, because the government, as the sole payer, controls what doctors can do and what they can charge.

Countries using the Beveridge Model, or variations on it, include its birthplace, Great Britain, as well as Italy, Spain, and most of Scandinavia. Hong Kong still has its own version of Beveridge-style national health care, because the populace simply refused to give it up when the Chinese took over the former British colony in 1997. The Beveridge Model, with government holding almost all the cards, is probably what Americans have in mind when they talk about "socialized medicine." Although this welfare-state approach to health care seems thoroughly European, the two purest examples of the Beveridge Model—or "socialized medicine"—are both found in the Western Hemisphere: Cuba and the U.S. Department of Veterans Affairs. In both of those systems, all the health care professionals work for the government in government-owned facilities, and patients generally receive no bills.

THE NATIONAL HEALTH INSURANCE MODEL

This system has elements of both Bismarck and Beveridge: The providers of health care are private, but the payer is a government-run insurance program that every citizen pays into. The national, or provincial, insurance plan collects monthly premiums and pays medical bills. Since there's no need for marketing, no expensive underwriting offices to deny claims, and no profit, these universal insurance programs tend to be cheaper and much simpler administratively than American-style private insurance. As a single payer covering everybody, the national insurance plan tends to have considerable market power to negotiate for lower prices. NHI countries also control costs by limiting the medical services they will pay for or by making patients wait to be treated.

The paradigmatic NHI system is Canada's; its universal application and its equal treatment for all satisfy Canada's national sense of community. Australia and some newly industrialized nations, including Taiwan and South Korea, have adopted variations on the NHI model.

THE OUT-OF-POCKET MODEL

Only the developed, industrialized nations—perhaps forty of the world's two hundred countries—have any established health care payment systems. Most of the nations on the planet are too poor and too disorganized to provide any kind of mass medical care. The basic rule in such countries is simple, and brutal: The rich get medical care; the poor stay sick or die. In poor countries, the well-to-do and the well-connected, such as government officials, can usually find a doctor and pay for care, at least in the big cities. In rural regions of Africa, India, China, and South America, hundreds of millions of people go their whole lives without ever seeing a doctor. They may have access, though, to a village healer (such as the one we'll meet in chapter 9) who practices traditional medicine using home-brewed remedies that may or may not be effective against disease.

A hallmark of these no-system countries is that most medical care is paid for by the patient, out of pocket, with no insurance or government plan to help. Generally, the world's poorest countries have the highest percentage of out-of-pocket payment for health. Out-of-pocket payments account for 91 percent of total health spending in Cambodia, 85 percent in India, and 73 percent in Egypt. In contrast, the figure for

Britain is 3 percent. The United States, with more than 45 million uninsured, ranks fairly high among wealthy countries on this scale, with 17 percent of health care costs funded by out-of-pocket payments.[1]

THESE FOUR MODELS SHOULD be fairly easy for Americans to understand, because we have elements of all of them in our convoluted national health care apparatus:

- **For most working people under sixty-five, we're Germany** or Japan. In standard Bismarck Model fashion, the worker and the employer share the premiums for a health insurance policy. The insurer picks up most of the tab for treatment, with the patient either making a co-payment or paying a percentage.

- **For Native Americans, military personnel, and veterans, we're Britain,** or Cuba. The VA and much of the Pentagon's Tri-Star system involve doctors who are government employees working in government-owned clinics and hospitals. Following the Beveridge Model, Americans in these systems never get a medical bill. The Indian Health Service also provides free care in government clinics.

- **For those over sixty-five, we're Canada.** U.S. Medicare is essentially a National Health Insurance scheme, with the near-universal participation and the low administrative costs that characterize such systems. Americans with end-stage renal disease, regardless of age, are also covered by Medicare; this group had enough political clout to get what it wanted from Congress, and the "dialysis community" opted for coverage under the government-run NHI system.

- **For the 45 million uninsured Americans, we're Cambodia,** or Burkina Faso, or rural India. These people have access to medical care if they can pay the bill out of pocket at the time of treatment, or if they're sick enough to be admitted to the emergency ward at a public hospital, or if they have access to a charity clinic.

- **And yet we're like no other country,** because the United States maintains so many separate systems for separate classes of people, and because it relies so heavily on for-profit private insurance plans to pay the bills. All the other countries have settled on one model for everybody, on the theory that this is simpler, cheaper, and fairer. With its fragmented array of providers and payers and overlapping systems, the U.S. health care system doesn't fit into any of the recognized models.

UNDERSTANDING THE four basic models significantly narrows down the global study of health care systems. When I set out looking for ideas and approaches we could borrow to fix American health care, I didn't have to go to two hundred different countries. I didn't even have to go to all thirty-six of the countries that rated higher than the United States when the World Health Organization compiled its rankings of the world's best health care systems. As admirable as medicine may be in places like San Marino (No. 11 on the WHO list) and Andorra (No. 21), it didn't seem particularly useful to study nations with populations smaller than Pittsburgh's.

Rather, I focused mainly on big countries with political, economic, and educational structures like ours: free-market democracies that have embraced the high-tech world. I wanted to see examples of each of the standard models: Bismarck, Beveridge, National Health Insurance, and Out-of-Pocket. I tried to choose countries that had faced, and tried to solve, the same basic problems facing our health care system, like an aging population and the rapidly escalating costs of modern medicine and drugs. And I wanted to visit health care systems that have been recognized, in the WHO study and other global surveys, as generally excellent. That way, I would find the world's best medical practices—and put my sore shoulder in good hands at the same time.

In the end, those criteria steered me to France, Germany, and Japan (all Bismarck) and to Britain (Beveridge) and Canada (NHI). I went to three Bismarck Model nations on the theory that this private-sector approach is the most familiar to most Americans and thus the most likely to be chosen as a model when America finally decides to provide universal health care. To see how things work in the out-of-pocket world, I set off for India as well, where Mrs. Rama predicted, accurately, that my right shoulder could be successfully treated.

But even if we found good ideas in those other countries, could the United States find the political will at home to use them? One basic political truth about American health care is that our system is strongly resistant to change. The vested interests that are doing well in the health business now—insurance companies, hospital chains, pharmaceutical companies—have blocked significant restructuring of our system.

But then, every industrialized democracy has vested interests that resist change. So I went to Switzerland and Taiwan, two countries that recently overcame the political hurdles and reformed their health care systems. The key lesson I took from those countries is that fundamental change would be easier to implement than our timid politicians seem to believe.

EVEN THOUGH I FOCUSED on fairly similar countries—rich, capitalist democracies—I found an enormous variety of systems, methods, and philosophies in the way health care is provided and paid for. I found lavish, chrome-plated hospitals and clinics, as well as spartan, bare-bones facilities. But common threads wove through all these systems, most of which made me optimistic about the prospects for major improvements in our own health care arrangements. If we could import these common principles from the other rich countries, our health care system would work better for patients, providers, payers, and the American economy.

COVERAGE

All the developed countries I looked at provide health coverage for every resident, old or young, rich or poor. This is the underlying moral principle of the health care system in every rich country—every one, that is, except the United States. Some Americans get great health care. Some, like Nikki White, get little or none. And these disparities have a racial element. Blacks and Hispanics are less likely than whites to get treatment for serious disease and more likely to die from the illness. A universal health care network, like those in place in Europe and East Asia, would eliminate this basic inequality in American life.

Coverage for everybody would be fairer for the American people, and it would be fairer for American employers that provide health insurance for their workers. Since many companies don't do that—and the number of companies opting out of the health insurance system is growing, because the premiums are so costly—the employers who do provide insurance face a cost disadvantage against their competitors. The 2010 health reform act provides subsidies to help small employers provide health coverage, but our system still penalizes employers who are decent enough to their workers to buy insurance.

Another aspect of fairness in the delivery of medical care concerns decisions about which drugs or treatments or technology can be used and which patients can get them—that is, the rationing of health care. In American political debates, "rationing" is treated as a bad word. In fact, every country rations care, including the United States, as Nikki White learned so painfully. A British health minister, John Reid, explained the concept to me with a simple phrase: "We cover every-body, but we don't cover everything."

The key questions: Who makes those access-to-treatment decisions, and how uniformly are they applied? Should the system spend its money to keep a ninety-five-year-old Alzheimer's patient alive until he's ninety-six? Should an ailing eighty-four-year-old get the same intensive treatment for breast cancer that is provided to an otherwise healthy forty-four-year-old? Should the health system, or the insurance plan, pay for Viagra? For Botox? In a health care system that offers universal coverage, these decisions tend to be made uniformly for everybody, often by a governmental body acting transparently. (The British government unit that makes these life-or-death decisions is called, with a nice irony, NICE, an acronym for National Institute for Health and Clinical Excellence.) In the United States, such decisions are made, often in secret, by scores of different insurance companies. One person may get coverage for a potentially life-saving operation, while the next person doesn't. This may be a boon to the person with the more generous insurance policy, but it's not particularly fair.

QUALITY

Even though they spend considerably less, the other industrialized countries produce better results, in terms of overall national health and longevity, than American medicine does. In the next chapter, we'll look at some studies that have made such comparisons.

COST

Many Americans are worried that a national health care system with universal coverage would be an expensive proposition for the

United States. In fact, a better-organized system, covering everybody, would almost certainly cut our health care costs—after all, every other rich nation's health care system is cheaper than ours. Americans also tend to believe that the private sector can run a medical system for less money than government can; all the evidence from around the world suggests the opposite.

Reducing our health care costs, in turn, would reduce the competitive disadvantage faced by American companies because of the health insurance coverage they have to provide for their employees. American auto executives argue that each luxury car produced in the United States—a Cadillac, for example, or a Lincoln—has about $2,500 of employee health care cost built into its price structure, while the figure for a competing car produced overseas is zero dollars.[2] That claim makes for a dramatic PowerPoint chart, but it's not accurate. Japanese and German automakers pay health insurance premiums for their workers, just as Ford and GM do. (In fact, Japanese companies often build and run hospitals for their workers; Toyota has several of them in Toyota City, just outside Nagoya.) Canadian companies, British companies, and others pay for their national health care program through payroll taxes and corporate income taxes. But because those foreign health care systems cost so much less to run than ours, foreign competitors pay far less for health coverage than American companies do.

CHOICE

Some national health care systems limit a patient's choices—of doctors, hospitals, treatments—in order to save money. American health insurance plans and Medicare do the same thing, with their "provider networks," "approved formularies," and so on. The striking fact is that many countries provide *more* choice than most Americans have. When my family lived in Britain, there was no predetermined "network" to restrict our choice of a family doctor; the National Health Service let us go just about anywhere. We picked the clinic that was right down the street, but we didn't have to. In France, it's a basic rule that patients can go to any doctor or any hospital they choose, anywhere in France. In Japan, too, all insurance plans are required to pay the bills of any doctor or clinic in the entire country; the patient, not the insurance plan, decides which doctor to use.

Some countries offer no choice in health insurance; you take the plan your employer, or your local government, provides. But in Germany, Switzerland, and the Netherlands, any resident can choose any insurance plan on the market—and change to a new plan on short notice. That's a wider choice of health insurance than any American has.

ONE OTHER CONSTANT I found under all models is that every country on earth faces difficult problems in providing medical care to its people. Nobody's system is perfect. There are health care horror stories in every wealthy country—and they're true. All national health systems, even those that do their job well, are fighting a desperate battle these days against rising costs. We live in a technological age, and technology—in the form of new miracle drugs, new medical devices (e.g., man-made shoulders), and new procedures—plays a huge role in modern medicine. This is unquestionably a good thing; people are living longer, healthier lives than they could have without these high-tech medical advances. But it is also an expensive thing. One result has been a seemingly endless round of "health care reform" proposals in the developed nations as governments look for ways to deal with increased medical expenses without denying their population the benefits of new medical breakthroughs. In every rich country, there is so much money floating through the health care system that some people can't resist the temptation to cheat. All the nations I visited have their share of frauds and scams on par with the American experience.

Bitter contention over health care and its financing is so common nowadays that the American economist Tsung-Mei Cheng has formulated, with tongue only partly in cheek, the Universal Laws of Health Care Systems:

1. "No matter how good the health care in a particular country, people will complain about it."
2. "No matter how much money is spent on health care, the doctors and hospitals will argue that it is not enough."
3. "The last reform always failed."[3]

Everywhere I went on my global quest, I found that Cheng's Universal Laws held true.

But for all their problems, the other industrialized countries tend to do better than the United States on basic measures of health system performance: coverage, quality, cost control, choice. This was the most surprising and infuriating discovery of my global quest—that the United States of America performs so poorly in this fundamental area of human life. In industry, finance, music, science, arts, academics, athletics, Americans can match or surpass any other country. Why can't we do that when it comes to health care? What are we doing wrong?

THREE

The Paradox

WE START WITH A PARADOX: AT THE BEGINNING OF THE twenty-first century, the United States of America is the most powerful, most innovative, and richest nation the planet has ever known. But while this great nation is strong, smart, and wealthy, it is not particularly healthy compared to other developed nations. When it comes to the essential task of providing health care for people, the mighty USA is a fourth-rate power.

This is particularly paradoxical because the American medical establishment boasts many assets that no other country can match. The United States has the best-educated doctors, nurses, and medical technicians of any nation. We have the best-equipped hospitals. American laboratories lead the world in medical research; American companies set the global standard in developing miracle drugs and advanced medical technology (like the titanium shoulder Dr. Ferlic recommended for me). If you walk along Main Street or through the mall in any American city, you will almost certainly pass people who would be dead if it weren't for the skill and dedication of some physician. This is the picture of American medicine conveyed by TV shows like *House* and *Grey's Anatomy*, where dedicated, highly trained professionals save a half-dozen lives each week before the first commercial break. For anyone with the money—or the insurance policy—to pay for it, American medical treatment ranks with the best on earth. That's why seriously rich people all over the world tend to board their private jets and race to some famous American clinic when they face a medical emergency. That's why, when I visited a sparkling new state-of-the-art hospital in Singapore, the sign outside said the facility was run by Duke University Medical School. The government of Singapore—an island nation floating off the Malay Peninsula in the South China Sea, about as far from North Carolina as you can get—decided that the best possible place to find medical expertise was in Durham, North Carolina, USA.

But the sad fact is, we've squandered this treasure. We've wasted our shining medical assets because of a health care payment system—or, more precisely, a crazy quilt of several overlapping and often conflicting systems—that prevents millions from receiving the treatment they need and that undermines the quality of care for millions more. The shortcomings of our system can be grouped into three basic problems: coverage, quality, and cost.

COVERAGE

Nikki White, the woman we met on the first page of this book, symbolizes the central moral flaw of U.S. health care: Our system doesn't cover everybody. All the other developed countries see to it that every person has a right to health care when necessary. We don't.

There are tens of millions of Americans who can't go to the doctor when they're sick, or don't take the pills that could keep them well, because they can't pay for the office visit or the prescription. Some

Americans get world-class, state-of-the-art treatment for a chronic disease, while other Americans die from the same disease for lack of treatment. In the richest country on earth, there are children going to bed at night with an earache, with a toothache, with an asthma attack that leaves them gasping for the next breath, because their parents don't dare face a doctor bill. In other developed countries, those sick children would see a doctor and get the medicine they need regardless of the family's income. In comparative studies of health system performance in twenty-three developed nations, the Commonwealth Fund, a private U.S. foundation dedicated to promoting a better U.S. health care system, ranked the USA last when it comes to providing universal access to medical care.[1] When the World Health Organization rated the national health care systems of 191 countries in terms of "fairness," the United States ranked fifty-fourth.[2] That put us slightly ahead of Chad and Rwanda, but just behind Bangladesh and the Maldives.

This gap in coverage is not just a moral issue; it has severe practical impacts. As we'll see shortly, the United States does poorly on common benchmarks like curing people who have curable diseases. A key reason is that millions of us can't get to the doctor for a cure. Americans die every day from medical problems like lupus, cervical cancer, and diabetes, which could have been cured, or at least controlled, with medical care. Of course American doctors know how to treat those ailments—but only if the sick person has access to treatment. The cohort of Americans who don't have health insurance on any given day numbers over 45 million (about 15 percent of the population). The health reform act passed in 2010 will reduce their number significantly, but we'll still have about 23 million people uninsured when the new law takes full effect. Americans who don't have enough money or enough insurance to buy medical care can sometimes go to the emergency room—but only if they're on the verge of death or in active labor. For the vast majority of sick people, the emergency room is not an option. Beyond that, you can't go down to the emergency room for the physical exam or the blood test or the breast palpitation that could head off some disease before it threatens your life. You can't go back to the ER to refill the prescription for the pills required to keep you alive. Nikki White couldn't go to the emergency room for the standard lupus treatments that would have given her a normal life span.

In addition to those who have no health insurance coverage, tens of millions of Americans have coverage so limited that they are not protected against any serious bill from a doctor or a hospital. For those Americans who are uninsured or underinsured, any bout with illness can be terrifying on two levels. In addition to the risk of disability or death due to the disease, there's the risk of financial ruin due to the medical and pharmaceutical bills. This is a uniquely American problem. When I was traveling the world on my quest, I asked the health ministry of each country how many citizens had declared bankruptcy in the past year because of medical bills. Generally, the officials responded to this question with a look of astonishment, as if I had asked how many flying saucers from Mars landed in the ministry's parking lot last week. How many people go bankrupt because of medical bills? In Britain, zero. In France, zero. In Japan, Germany, the Netherlands, Canada, Switzerland: zero. In the United States, according to a joint study by Harvard Law School and Harvard Medical School, the annual figure is around 700,000.[3]

QUALITY

For all the money America spends on health care, our health outcomes are worse on many basic measures than those in countries that spend much less.

Some Americans get the world's best medical care (some Singaporeans do, too, by buying it from us). Overall, though, the quality of care provided by the U.S. medical system is mediocre by global standards.

For all its organizational problems, I had thought that hands-on American medicine was top-notch. But comparative studies repeatedly demonstrate that this is not so.

One classic benchmark for a national medical system is "avoidable mortality"—that is, how well a country does at curing diseases that are curable. A 2008 report by the Commonwealth Fund, "Deaths Before Age 75 from Conditions That Are at Least Partially Modifiable with Effective Medical Care," concluded that the United States is the worst of the developed countries on this measure. Among nineteen wealthy countries, the United States ranked nineteenth in curing people who could be cured with decent care. (However, we did better than any of the world's poor countries.) The number of people under seventy-five who die from curable illness was almost twice as high in the United States as in the countries that do the best on this measure: France, Japan, and Spain.[4]

Another way to measure the quality of medical treatment is to compare the survival rate from major diseases. On this score, too, the United States generally comes out badly in comparison to other rich countries. A Commonwealth Fund study of nine developed countries between 2001 and 2004[5] showed that Americans diagnosed with asthma die sooner than their counterparts in seven of the countries. (British asthmatics fared even worse than Americans did.) Americans with diabetes die younger than diabetics in any of the other countries. After kidney transplants, Americans have the worst survival rate. And if you've been thinking about having major surgery in the United States, here's a statistic to ponder: Among those nine rich nations, the per-capita rate of "Deaths Due to Surgical or Medical Mishaps" was the highest by far in the USA. For some particular ailments, U.S. medicine tops the world. America's five-year survival rate for women diagnosed with breast cancer was the best of the nine countries in this study. But overall, we lag the other rich countries in treating many of the diseases that medicine knows how to treat.

In terms of life expectancy—how many years the average newborn baby is likely to live—the United States ranks below most European countries and rich East Asian countries like Japan, Taiwan, and Singapore. But our country's score here is skewed somewhat, because more people die young in America than in other rich countries. For those of us who are adults, and wondering how many good years we've got left, the medical researchers have a more relevant benchmark: "healthy life expectancy at age sixty." That predicts not just how many more years a sixty-year-old can expect to live, but how long she can expect to feel pretty good; that is, how long she can expect to live before the onset of predictable ailments of the aged, such as Alzheimer's disease and rheumatoid arthritis. Since this is largely a function of medical care, any country's score on "healthy life expectancy at age sixty" turns out to be a pretty good measure of that country's medical system. And on this one, too, we're in the basement. Among twenty-three countries in a 2006 survey by the Commonwealth Fund, the United States was tied for last. (Japan came in first.)[6]

Anyone reading this book has obviously lived long enough to learn to read. Some Americans don't get that far. Perhaps the most tragic indicator of America's troubled health care system is the number of newborns who die each year. This statistic is called infant mortality, or neonatal death. It generally refers to babies who die within one year of birth. To me, that seems the most painful thing that could ever happen: The expectant parents go through the anticipation and sheer joy of watching their baby develop in the womb, enter the world, join the family—and then have to bury a tiny corpse a few weeks later. Surely any decent health care system would develop effective mechanisms to avoid neonatal death. But out of twenty-three wealthy countries, the American health care system ranks dead last when it comes to keeping newborns alive. Our rate of infant mortality is more than twice as high as the rate in the top-ranked countries, Sweden and Japan.[7] A key reason, as we'll see in later chapters, is that other rich countries offer free prenatal and neonatal care for every mother and every baby. This is costly—but it's much less expensive, both economically and emotionally, than the heroic surgical efforts used in the United States to save threatened infants.

INFANT MORTALITY RATES, 2008

Country	Deaths per 1,000 births
Sweden	2.76
Japan	2.8
Norway	3.64
France	3.41
Germany	4.08
Switzerland	4.2
Canada	4.63
UK	5.01
Cuba	6.04
United States	6.37

Source: CIA World Factbook, 2009.

COST

As we've seen already, the United States is by far the world's biggest spender on health care. Whether measured as a percentage of the nation's GDP or as per-capita spending, we pour roughly twice as much into medicine as other rich countries do. Given what we've just read about coverage and quality, that raises an obvious question: If we're getting only fair-to-middling performance from a system that leaves tens of millions of people without reliable health care, why are we paying more than anybody else? Why does American health care cost so much?

One reason (though not the main one) is that American health care "providers"—doctors, nurses, hospitals, drug companies—make more money for what they do than their counterparts overseas do. When Americans fill a prescription, the price is routinely twice as much—sometimes ten times as much—as a Briton or a German would pay for precisely the same pills made in the same factory. Our standard image of a physician—fairly accurate, although there are exceptions—depicts someone who lives in the fancy suburb and drives a Lexus to the best country club after work. But that's not the standard picture of a doctor's life in other countries. Christina von Köckritz, the charming, intelligent German general practitioner we'll meet in chapter 5, complained to me about her economic status, noting that she was a "pauper" compared to her peers in the United States. "They work no more than I do, but they make money two times, three times as much," she told me. Judging from average income data for doctors in the two countries, she's about right.

But these comparisons don't take us very far. It's true that Frau Doktor von Köckritz earns a lot less in annual income than an American doctor would expect to take in. But there are other considerations. Newly minted American doctors generally owe student loans of $100,000 or more on the day they receive their M.D. degrees. Dr. Von Köckritz's entire higher education was free. She considers that perfectly normal—and in Europe, it is. Dr. Von Köckritz told me that she pays about 1,000 per year ($1,400) for malpractice insurance, and she doubts that she would ever be sued. Her American counterpart could be paying a hundred times as much for malpractice insurance, depending on the state, and will likely be sued several times during her career.

In any case, the big money providers earn is not the major cause of high medical spending in the United States. Most economists who study this question have concluded that lower fees and prices would save Americans something, but not much. If we cut the average American physician's pay to European levels, and told the drug companies they can't charge more for Lipitor in the United States than they do in the UK, there would be savings, but not nearly enough to bring our medical spending down to the levels in the rest of the developed world.

Another widely cited culprit for our high medical costs—Americans' penchant for filing malpractice lawsuits against their doctors—also turns out to be a minor contributor to overall costs. If we banned malpractice suits, it would relieve stress on doctors and perhaps eliminate some unnecessary tests that doctors order only as a defensive measure in case they are ever sued. But it wouldn't save the health care system a lot of money. Economists who study this topic say that the nation's total malpractice bill, including insurance premiums, big-dollar verdicts, and defensive medicine, adds only 1 percent to our total health care costs.[8] Several states have imposed strict limits on malpractice damage awards, but the impact on costs has been minimal. Texas passed the toughest malpractice controls in the country, but health care costs in Texas have risen faster than the national average, despite that law.[9]

Rather, the major reasons our national medical bill is so much higher than any other country's are two things that the United States does differently from every other country: the way we manage health insurance and the complexity of our health care system.

The United States is the only developed country that relies on profit-making health insurance companies to pay for essential and elective care. About 80 percent of non-elderly Americans have health insurance; generally they get it through the job, with the employer paying part of the premium as well. The monthly premium goes toward paying the worker's medical bills, but the insurance firms also soak up a significant share of the premium dollar to cover the costs of marketing, underwriting, and administration, as well as their profit. Economists agree that this is about the most expensive possible way to pay for a nation's health care. That's why, as we'll see throughout this book, all the other developed countries have decided that basic health insurance must be a nonprofit operation. In those countries, the insurance plans—sometimes run by government, sometimes private entities—exist only to pay people's medical bills, not to provide dividends for investors.

It's revealing that, in the lingo of the U.S. health insurance industry, the money paid to doctors, hospitals, and pharmacies for treatment of insured patients is referred to as "medical loss." That is, when health insurance actually pays for somebody's health care, the industry considers it a loss. (Health insurance executives explain that "loss ratio" is a technical term borrowed from the fire and casualty insurance business.) Insurance executives, securities analysts, and the business media carefully watch each company's medical loss ratio to make sure that the actual medical payments don't eat too deeply into administrative costs and profits. According to their filings with the Securities and Exchange Commission, most for-profit insurance companies maintain a medical loss ratio of about 80 percent, which is to say that 20 cents of every dollar people pay in premiums for health insurance doesn't buy any health care.[10] If a health insurance company consistently spent much more than 80 percent of its money on actual health care, its stock would plummet and its CEO would be axed. Under enormous pressure, the insurance industry agreed to provisions in the health reform act of 2010 that will eventually limit their administrative costs for certain plans to 20 percent (and in some cases, 15 percent) of premium income. But even with these new strictures, the U.S. private insurers will still be the least efficient health care payers anywhere.

Every organization, public or private, business or charity, has administrative costs. But the U.S. private insurance industry has the highest administrative costs of any health care payer in the world. Americans tend to believe that the private sector can manage any type of business better than government can. This is not the case, though, when it comes to health insurance. Medicare, the government-run single-payer system created by Congress in 1965 to pay for basic health care for the elderly, has administrative costs of about 3 percent; the single-payer government systems run by different provinces in Canada have about the same. Britain's National Health Service, a system where government both provides and pays for health care, has administrative costs of 5 percent.

American health insurance also differs from the other countries on the question of "guaranteed issue." In other developed countries, health insurance plans are required by law to guarantee coverage for anybody. American insurance firms, though, are allowed to pick and choose their customers. They pour large sums of money into efforts to cherry-pick the right customers and avoid the wrong ones. That way, they can avoid selling health insurance to the people who need the most health care—and are the most expensive to cover.[11] The United States is the only developed country that allows insurance companies to refuse coverage to people for fear that they might get sick.

The American insurers point out—and they're right—that they have to pick and choose their customers to avoid a problem known as "adverse selection." That term refers to people who refuse to buy health insurance when they're healthy but go shopping for a plan after they've been diagnosed with a serious disease. If an insurance company had to sell coverage to all those people, it would quickly face claims in excess of the premiums it took in. The solution to adverse selection is to mandate that everybody pay for health insurance, through either a private company or a government program. That requirement is known as the "individual mandate," and it is a necessary corollary to "guaranteed issue." If insurance companies have to cover everybody who applies, they need to have everybody in the insurance pool to cover the costs. All other developed countries require both "guaranteed issue" and the "individual mandate."

In the 2010 health reform act, Congress followed the international models and required both guaranteed issue and the individual mandate for American health insurance. But the mandate was phased in gradually and was challenged in a highly politicized lawsuit by nineteen state attorneys general. Consequently, it will take several years at least before these two elements of health insurance—standard operating procedure in other rich countires—become standard in the United States.

Insurers also do their best to restrict payments for the people they do cover. Anybody who has had the dubious pleasure of submitting claims to an American health insurance company probably knows that the insurance firms spend a lot of time and money figuring out how to avoid paying medical bills. They hire armies of adjusters and investigators to go through submitted claims looking for reasons to deny payment; it is cheaper to send out a form letter saying "claim denied" than to write a check to the doctor or the patient. In other developed countries, insurers are required to pay every claim. But U.S. insurance companies deny about 30 percent of all claims, although some of these are eventually paid through an appeal process.[11] The reasons cited for denying valid claims can be ingenious. When our family lived in Japan, the friendly adjusters at Prudential used to deny our claims for medical or dental care on the grounds that the bills we submitted were denominated in yen. Somebody at Prudential had determined that the Japanese yen was a foreign currency; that violated the rules. My company later switched our health insurance to Aetna, which employed a similar dodge: The adjuster said she couldn't pay our claims because she couldn't call the doctor's office to verify the bills. It seems that Aetna had a phone system for its adjusters that didn't allow international calls. So naturally, all our claims had to be denied.

The 2010 reform act includes no significant regulation of claim payments, so insurers will still be able to deny claims on any grounds they choose. But the new law did prohibit some of the most reprehensible practices of the U.S. insurance industry. Beginning in the fall of 2010, health insurers will no longer be able to use the gambit known as "recission," a cruel legal maneuver they employed to cancel the policies of a customer who had a serious accident or contracted a major disease so that the patient, not the insurance company, would get stuck with the bills. And insurers will no longer be able to set an arbitrary limit on payments, another tool they invented to shift medical bills from the insurance company to the patient.

But the new law does not directly confront another harsh anomaly of U.S. health insurance: Unlike people in other rich countries, Americans under sixty-five can't get health insurance that is permanent. If you leave your job, voluntarily or otherwise, you lose your insurance. No other country uses that model, because it hits the victim with a double whammy. She not only loses most of her income, but she loses her family's insurance coverage precisely at the moment when she is most economically vulnerable. In the rest of the world, this is considered unbelievably cruel. "Excuse me, Mr. Reid, but I don't understand your approach to health care," a junior minister in Sweden's health department said to me. "It seems to me that your country takes away the insurance when people most need it." Of all the mysterious nooks and crannies of U.S. health policy, the rule that takes away insurance coverage from those most in need may be the hardest to justify. In France, Germany, Japan, etc., people get health insurance as a benefit of employment, but the coverage continues if the job ends. Government pays the premium until the unlucky employee can get back to work. She may not have a job, but she can still afford to take her sick child to the doctor.

As we'll see in later chapters, other countries do allow health insurance companies to make a profit on some supplemental policies—but not on the basic coverage plan available to everybody. In France, some elderly people buy insurance to get them a spot in an upscale nursing home. In Britain, private insurance pays for cosmetic surgery and for some other operations, like cataract repair and knee replacements—not to mention my "total shoulder arthroplasty"—that the free National Health Service doesn't usually offer. British patients can also use private insurance to get an earlier appointment with a specialist and thus avoid the queues in the NHS. In India, insurance covers the services of astrologers like Mrs. Rama. But no other country relies on for-profit insurance companies to pay for basic health care. As we'll see in chapter 10, Switzerland used to have U.S.-style, profit-making health insurance, but the Swiss dropped that system on the theory that health insurance has to be nonprofit in order to do its job. Switzerland still has private health insurance companies; but the firms can't make a profit on the basic coverage package, and they have to cover everybody, regardless of "adverse selection" concerns.[13]

The second major anomaly of the U.S. system—the flaw that forces us to spend more than any other country on health—is sheer complexity. We have developed, more or less by accident, the most fragmented health care system in the developed world, with "providers" sending bills to a vast array of different payers.

All the other developed countries have settled on one health care system for everybody; that means every patient is treated equally, and there's one set of rules governing treatment and payment. (Some countries have a separate military medical system for soldiers overseas, but as soon as those soldiers get home, they go into the national system with everybody else.) The United States, in contrast, is a crazy quilt of different payment systems. There's one system for Americans over sixty-five. There's one for military personnel, and a different one for veterans. There's a separate system for Native Americans and yet another for people with end-stage renal failure. There's one system for Americans under sixteen living in poor families and a different one for people over sixteen in poor families. Members of Congress have provided themselves with a terrific health care system of their own, which gives them a choice among numerous private insurance plans plus the option to be treated in military medical centers like Bethesda Naval Hospital. And there are scores, perhaps hundreds, of different private insurance plans. Each paying entity has its own distinct rules about what care it will pay for and how much it will pay. Quite often, neither the buyer (the patient) nor the seller (the doctor) knows how much a particular treatment costs. When Dr. Ferlic recommended a man-made shoulder to replace my aching joint, I asked him how much it would cost. The doctor, after all, was going to perform the surgery and issue a bill, so I assumed he would know the price. Not a chance. "I couldn't possibly answer that," he said frankly. "That's determined by your insurance company, and they all have different payment schedules. There are even different payments for different insurance plans from the same company."

The presence of countless different payers and fee schedules drives another unique feature of American health care: the cost shift. Medical providers—doctors, hospitals, labs—naturally try to shift costs toward the highest payer. If Medicare, with its recurrent budget problems, cuts the fee it pays a hospital for a particular procedure, the hospital will raise the price for other payers to make up the difference. That's another reason why the same operation in the same hospital on the same day can have ten different prices, depending on who is paying.

The administrative patchwork makes everything about American medicine more complex and more expensive than it needs to be. A British hospital, a Taiwanese hospice, or a Canadian clinic will deal with one paying entity and one standard payment schedule. When you go to the doctor in France, the standard fee schedule for each potential treatment is posted on the wall, showing exactly what the bill will be and how much of it the insurance plan will cover. U.S. hospitals, in contrast, routinely deal with twenty, fifty, or a hundred different public and private payers. Even a neighborhood doctor's office, with three or four family physicians and four nurses, will have a corps of four to

THE WALL STREET JOURNAL

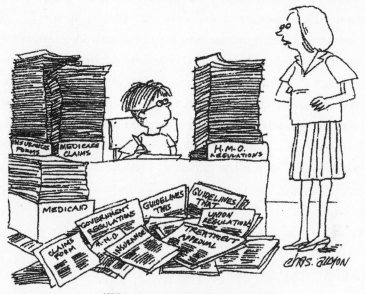

**"How many times have I told
you not to play doctor?"**

eight people in the back room just to handle the billing. Not surprisingly, one of the fastest-growing aspects of the American health care industry is the booming business for "compilers," middlemen who compile the bills that doctors submit and then shuttle them through the payment system. This makes life easier for doctors, but at a price: It adds an extra level of complexity and yet another layer of bills to the overall cost of American medicine. The *Wall Street Journal* neatly summarized the general state of affairs in a cartoon that was thumbtacked to the wall in just about every American doctor's office.

"Like other observers," noted the prominent health care economist Henry Aaron, of the Brookings Institution, "I look at the U.S. health care program and see an administrative monstrosity, a truly bizarre mélange of thousands of payers with payment systems that differ for no socially beneficial reason, as well as staggeringly complex public systems with mind-boggling administered prices and other rules expressing distinctions that can only be regarded as weird."[14] The administrative monstrosity we have built costs us a lot of money—by far the highest administrative costs of any health care system on earth. The U.S. Government Accountability Office concluded that if the country could get the administrative costs of its medical system down to the Canadian level, the money saved would be enough to pay for health care for all the Americans who are uninsured.

But the 2010 reform law did little to reduce the fragmentation of American health care; if anything, it will give us a system that is even more complex.

THE U.S. HEALTH CARE system's troubles with quality, coverage, and cost control are well-known in the rest of the developed world. When health industry executives, public health officials, or health care economists gather for international meetings, bashing the U.S. system is a standard agenda item. "You get used to it after a while," says Princeton professor Uwe E. Reinhardt, one of the most distinguished American economists in the field. "Economists love to disagree, and they argue about everything. But at these conferences, the one thing they all agree on is that the American system is a huge mess. In health care, the United States has become the bogeyman of the world."

In the same way, the American health care system is constantly invoked by politicians around the world as a dangerous jungle to be avoided at all costs. Whenever some aspect of a nation's health care system is criticized, the all-purpose response from those in power is "At least we're not as bad as the Americans." I saw this dynamic at work over and over when we lived in Britain. Each week in the British Parliament, the prime minister has to face a barrage of inquiries and insults known as Prime Minister's Questions. Almost every week, somebody from one of the opposition parties complains about the

National Health Service: Doctors are underpaid. Hospitals are leaky and crumbling. Patients have to wait months or even years for surgery. Something Must Be Done! In reply, the prime minister—both Tony Blair and his successor, Gordon Brown, used this gambit—goes on the attack. "The honorable gentleman opposite," the PM declares, "clearly hopes to turn our health care system into a profit-making corporate enterprise as the Americans have done. This we will never do!" Of course Blair and Brown both know that nobody in Britain has any intention of ditching the beloved National Health Service and replacing it with American-style medicine. But the mere invocation of that idea is an effective way to end the argument.

I don't think that Americans are any more willing to ditch our own health care system and replace it wholesale with a British or German or Canadian model. But there are useful approaches, ideas, and techniques we could learn from health care systems that are fairer, cheaper, and more effective than ours. That was the impulse behind my global quest: to look at the world's best systems and see if they had useful lessons for us. So my sore shoulder and I hit the road, looking for good ideas for managing a nation's health care. But where to begin? Just as Dwight D. Eisenhower copied the world's best highways, I decided to start my quest with the world's best health care system. So I began with the nation that stands at No. 1 in the World Health Organization's ranking, the most comprehensive comparative study of national health care systems ever undertaken. And that's what led me to a tiny, spartan medical office just down the street from the rococo splendor of the Palace of Versailles.

FOUR

France: The Vital Card

DR. BERTRAND TAMALET'S HANDSOME, YOUTHFUL FACE spread into a broad smile of recognition, as if he had just come upon a cherished old acquaintance he hadn't seen in years. In a sense, that's just what happened. As soon as Dr. Tamalet put the X-ray of my right shoulder up on the light box in his tiny office, he positively beamed with pride and delight. As an orthopedist, he instantly identified the type of surgical repair I had received at Bethesda Naval Hospital three decades earlier (the big stainless-steel screw holding my shoulder together tends to be a dead giveaway). As a Frenchman, he enjoyed a deep chauvinistic glow, because that particular shoulder operation, using a large screw to stabilize the injured joint, was pioneered by a French orthopedic surgeon, Dr. Maurice Latarjet, and later adopted by other orthopods around the world—including, obviously, the surgeons at Bethesda. "You had the Latarjet procedure!" the smiling doctor said with a burst of patriotic fervor. "We developed that one, you know. It's a French operation. And I can see that it has held up quite well over all these years."

As a matter of fact, I had not known about the national origin of my shoulder operation; my doctors back home called it a Bristow procedure, after the orthopedist who popularized the surgery in the States. (I subsequently did some research in the medical libraries and found that the standard texts on shoulder surgery do in fact refer to the French contribution. In the United States the operation is called the Bristow-Latarjet procedure. In France, naturally, it's Latarjet-Bristow.) But the discovery of a Frenchified shoulder in his American patient prompted the friendly, talkative Dr. Tamalet to launch into a detailed history of shoulder orthopedics in France. It is, to be fair, a distinguished history. By all accounts—even the Americans agree on this point—it was a French orthopedist who implanted the world's first man-made joint. Accordingly, anyone who is walking around pain-free on an artificial knee or hip owes a debt of gratitude to Dr. Jules Émile Péan and the bright idea he hit upon in March of 1892.

Dr. Péan was treating a thirty-seven-year-old baker who had come to the Hôpital Saint-Louis in Paris with a severe infection due to tuberculosis. The patient's shoulder was being eaten away by the disease. All the experts agreed on the remedy: immediate amputation, before the infection could spread. The patient steadfastly refused. Confronted by a stubborn patient facing almost certain death, Péan came up with a radical new treatment, never tried before: an artificial joint. He cut out the baker's infected ball-and-socket joint and replaced the shoulder with a shaft of platinum, topped by a black rubber ball coated with wax. Two metal loops encircling the waxed ball took the place of the socket. When the incision was closed, the patient walked back to his bakery, taking with him history's first total joint replacement. (It would be forty-two more years before doctors got around to a total hip replacement.) This first-ever "total shoulder arthroplasty" was a stunning success. The baker's body did not reject this alien implant, and the man-made shoulder worked well. Dr. Péan, having saved his patient's life and livelihood with a revolutionary idea, became the toast of

Parisian medicine. Henri de Toulouse-Lautrec painted a heroic portrait of the famous doctor, showing Péan as he cut deeply into a patient's damaged shoulder. The historic man-made shoulder, removed from the patient two years later, was presented to the Smithsonian Institution and can be seen today at the National Museum of Health and Medicine[1] in Washington, D.C.

Dr. Tamalet related this surgical history as we sat in his *cabinet médicale* on the rue Saint Adelaïde in a fairly grimy section of Versailles, southwest of Paris. We were barely three miles from the Sun King's spectacular palace, but there was nothing palatial about the doctor's office. It was a clean but austere rectangle of a place with an old linoleum floor and plain plaster walls, as narrow and drab as a single room in some fleabag hotel. It featured an examining table for patients to lie on and a couple of small wooden desks adorned with plastic models of the shoulder and spinal column. There was a computer screen and a keyboard on one of the desks and a light box mounted on the wall where the doctor could look at his patients' X-rays. A few doors down the hall of the dingy office building was the doctor's waiting room, a closet-sized space with four folding chairs, no table, no magazines, and nothing on the gray walls except a detailed chart showing precisely how much Dr. Tamalet would charge, and how much the national insurance plan would reimburse, for each form of treatment. My visit, a "consultation for joint pain or stiffness," was priced at 26, or $33.80. Patients were expected to pay this fee at the time of the visit, and the insurance would reimburse the patient about 70 percent of the fee, or $24. In other words, a visit to an orthopedic specialist would cost about $10 out of pocket. Back home, a "consultation for joint pain and stiffness" would cost me roughly four times as much—and considerably more if my insurance company denied the claim and stuck me with the whole bill.

These spartan surroundings and bargain-basement prices are fairly typical of French medicine. Although the French spend more on health care than most other European countries—and they worry incessantly about the cost of care—they are not spending much of that money to compensate doctors or hospitals. A physician's income, even in the ritziest Paris arrondissement, is a fraction of what a similarly situated doctor in the United States would make. As a result, French doctors and hospitals tend to be frugal when it comes to furnishings and ambience. Another way in which Dr. Tamalet's office was emblematic of French medicine was that lengthy price chart on the wall. In sharp contrast to American practice, French patients are informed up front, down to the last hundredth of a euro, how much they will pay for each medical procedure and how much they will get back from insurance. There was also something missing from the office, at least to American eyes. This doctor's office had no file cabinets or bookshelves loaded with patients' medical records and bills. How could you run a medical practice without files, and without bills?

There was one thing more in Dr. Tamalet's office that I had come to recognize as standard equipment in all French medical facilities: a green and gold sign that read: NOUS ACCEPTONS LA CARTE VITALE—"We accept the *carte vitale*." In a way, that promise was the most predictable, and the most important, element of the French health care system. For me, the *carte vitale*—a green plastic credit card with a small gold memory chip in the middle, the central administrative tool of French medicine—became a symbol of what the French have achieved in designing a health care system to treat the nation's 61 million residents.

They've achieved a lot. Whether or not you agree with the World Health Organization's conclusion that France has the world's No. 1 health care system, all the statistics on national health suggest that France rates near the top of the global rankings. France does a better job than almost any other country both in encouraging health and in treating those who get sick. As noted earlier, France has the best performance of any nation on a key measure, "Mortality Amenable to Health Care"—which is to say, the French medical system does the best job of curing people whose diseases are curable.[2] The French rank near the top—and sharply higher than the United States—on standard health measures like Disability-Adjusted Life Expectancy (DALE), infant mortality, and life expectancy among adults. (An average sixty-year-old Frenchwoman can expect to live in good health for a further twenty years and three months; a sixty-year-old American female will average another seventeen years and eleven months of healthy life.)[3] The French health insurance system covers every resident of France and guarantees everyone a roughly equal level of treatment. France has more doctors per capita than the United States and more hospital beds. The French go to the doctor about eight times per year, on average, compared to five visits for Americans; the average Frenchman takes more pills and shots than Americans do. Continuing the tradition of doctors Péan and Latarjet, the French are significant innovators in health care and pharmaceuticals. In short, the French are big consumers of medicine, and they get a high-quality product. Yet France pays less than we do for health care.

France's health care system is a variation on the Bismarck Model, a system that would be familiar to Americans. It is not "socialized medicine." Rather, it is largely a system of private doctors treating patients who buy health insurance—from a government health plan, and from private insurers—to cover most of the cost. As in the United States, most French doctors are in the private sector and charge patients on a fee-for-service basis; there's a specific charge for each office visit, injection, X-ray, and so on. As in the United States, the French buy health insurance through the job, with the employer and the worker splitting the cost; the monthly premium is withheld from the worker's paycheck. As in the United States, patients generally have to pay a fee, or co-pay, at the time of treatment; unlike the United States, the French patient will later have most or all of this co-pay reimbursed by the insurance fund. As in the United States, there are both public and private hospitals; the French for-profit hospitals tend to specialize in certain illnesses and procedures.

For the most part, French workers don't have a choice of health insurance plans; they get the one that was set up for their line of work, or their geographic region, and stick with it for life.

But there are also major differences with the United States, particularly when it comes to health insurance. Because the insurance plans—the *caisses d'assurance maladie,* or "sickness insurance funds"—are nonprofit entities, their main concern is not providing a return to investors but, rather, paying for people's health care. Consequently, the French system eliminates some aspects of health insurance that Americans hate the most. French insurance funds can't turn you down for coverage, regardless of preexisting conditions. They can't terminate your coverage when you lose or change your job. (When a French worker loses her job, she keeps the same insurance plan; the government pays the employer's share of the premium.) They can't deny a claim; once the doctor submits a bill, insurance has to pay it. There's no deductible; French insurance pays from the first euro billed. The long delays in reimbursement that are common for American insurance companies are illegal in France. Doctors and hospitals are generally paid within a week, and the patients must be reimbursed for their costs at the end of each month. Since the French insurance funds don't spend any money on marketing, on filtering out unwelcome customers, on reviewing and denying claims, or on paying dividends to stockholders, they are significantly more efficient businesses than American insurance companies. As we saw in chapter 3, the profit-making health insurance giants in the United States generally spend about 20 percent of all premium income on administrative expenses; the French insurance plans routinely keep administrative costs below 5 percent.[4]

As a general rule, the French don't have to wait in line to see a general practitioner or a specialist; waiting times are usually about the same as those for people with insurance in the United States. A key exception here is pediatricians, who are in short supply in France. That shortage disturbed a friend of mine in the north Paris suburb of Bondy, who had to wait until her son was six weeks old before she could get an appointment with his pediatrician. As is standard in France, a postnatal nurse came to visit mother and child at home several times in the first weeks after the birth, for free. "And that was good," the new mom told me, "but I wanted Samuel to meet his doctor!"

There's almost no limitation on a patient's choice in France. There's no such thing as the "in-network" and "out-of-network" lists developed by U.S. insurance companies; under French law, every health facility is "in-network." Any patient can go to any doctor, any specialist, any surgeon, and any hospital or clinic in the whole country, and the insurance system must pay the bill. If you feel sick, you can call an ambulance to take you to the doctor or hospital of your choice—for free. The French don't have the "gatekeeper" system, common in the United States and several other countries, in which you have to get a referral from a general practitioner before you can go to a specialist. The French tried to establish the gatekeeper process in 1997—it tends to save money for the system as a whole, because GPs can filter out some problems that don't need an expensive specialist's care—but the public rebelled against this limitation on free choice. With the streets of Paris blocked by furious demonstrations of patients and doctors, the government caved, reaffirming the right of any French patient to see any specialist, anytime.

And France achieves all that at a reasonable cost. Of course, the French don't consider their system cheap; their planners and politicians see only that nearby countries like Britain, Sweden, Italy, Spain, and the Netherlands all spend less on health care than France does. This has spawned repeated campaigns for health care reform over the years. Compared to the amount of money the U.S. health care system burns through each year, though, France's system looks like a bargain. France spends about $3,165 per capita each year for a health insurance system that covers everybody; the United States spends more than $7,000 per capita and leaves tens of millions without coverage. France's spending runs just under 10 percent of its total national wealth (as measured by gross domestic product); the United States is spending about 17 percent of GDP on health care.[5] A study by the Bank of America in 2006 concluded that if we Americans could get our health care spending down to the French level—say, 10 percent of GDP—we would save about $600 billion annually.[6] In the U.S. system, even with its built-in inefficiencies, that saving would meet the basic health care needs of all the Americans who are currently uninsured.

France's health insurance system, based on the "sickness funds" of the classic Bismarck Model, began in 1928 with a fund that covered only low-wage workers in certain industries. The egalitarian impulse in French society demanded that others get the same kind of benefit, and the system gradually expanded to cover every resident of France (although it wasn't until 2000 that the final 1 percent of the population got coverage). Today, everybody must belong to a health insurance fund; it's illegal to opt out, no matter how healthy you think you are. An employed or retired person gets coverage through his job, with the employer paying most of the cost; the worker's premium is withheld from his paycheck or pension. The unemployed must be covered as well, but the government pays the premium for them. There are three main insurance funds—one for salaried workers, one for farmworkers, and one for professionals and the self-employed—and eleven smaller ones covering a few specific industries. Premiums are dirt cheap, particularly for the employee. A single person making $20,000 per year paid $12.25 per month in 2007; her employer's share of the monthly premium was $208.

In addition to this required insurance, the French can also buy supplemental health insurance, either from nonprofit cooperatives (*mutuelles*) or from for-profit insurance companies; because this coverage is even cheaper than the sickness funds, almost 90 percent of workers buy it. The private insurance helps pay for the share of the co-pays that the sickness funds don't reimburse. It's also used like "Medi-gap" insurance in the United States to pay for treatment the mandatory policies don't cover, like face-lifts and tummy-tucks. For example, the basic package from the sickness funds does not cover treatment for the ailment delicately labeled "erectile dysfunction"—after all, it's a basic fact of life that lusty Frenchmen don't need artificial assistance in this area. For some strange reason, though, a lot of Frenchmen still take Viagra, and they use supplemental insurance to help cover the cost.

On paper, therefore, France is a multipayer health care system, with fourteen different sickness funds and a cluster of supplemental plans paying doctors and providers. In practice, France acts like a single-payer system, because the national Health Ministry essentially dictates what providers can charge for most types of treatment and what price will be paid for each prescription. Just as Aetna and UnitedHealth negotiate with doctors, hospitals, and drug companies to set fees in the United States, the French government negotiates, on behalf of the big sickness funds, with doctors, hospitals, and drug companies. The difference is that the French negotiations are completely transparent. That's why you see a highly detailed list of authorized fees in the waiting room when you go to the doctor in France. Most French doctors belong to a labor union, and these unions do the negotiating on behalf of the physicians. As with most other labor unions in France, the physicians' unions tend to do their negotiating on the picket line. Leading health economists complain that this amounts to "making health care policy through strikes." This charge is accurate. But then, a lot of policy disputes in France are resolved through strikes.

The people of France are proud of their health care system; just about every French citizen seems to know that the World Health Organization rated their country best in the world for "Overall Health System Attainment." Some Frenchmen take this achievement as further proof—as if any were needed—that France is superior to the planet's other countries. The WHO rating "reinforced the public view that France had an excellent" health system, said Professor Jean de Kervasdoué, a health economist in Paris. "The French despise the inequitable American system and could not bear to think of anything like British waiting lists or any other overt method of rationing."[7] And yet these same French are constantly changing their system; there were major reforms in 1996, 1997, 2000, and 2004. This makes France a mirror image of the United States when it comes to health care: Americans strongly dislike their national health care system, but find it enormously difficult to make changes; the French are highly satisfied with their system, but change it all the time. France is living proof of the first of the Universal Laws of Health Care Systems we ran across in chapter 2: "No matter how good the health care in a particular country, people will complain about it."

Sometimes the changes result from public concern about the quality of French medical care. When about fifteen thousand elderly French people died during an intense heat wave in August 2003, the politicians demanded improvement in ambulance services and emergency rooms. Most of the recent complaints, though, have been driven by a single concern: money. The French are convinced that their health care system is simply too expensive to sustain. Just about everybody involved in health policy in France tends to say the same thing: "Our health care system costs too much." Most of the sickness funds run up operating deficits year after year. The last major round of reforms, in 2004, gave the national government even more control over prices and procedures. The result is that the sickness funds, which began as more or less independent health insurance plans, now operate more like branches of the Health Ministry, with their rules and fees controlled by bureaucrats in Paris. The 2004 law also made yet another effort to employ general practitioners as gatekeepers in order to cut the fees owed to specialists. This was done in the gentlest possible way: Under the new arrangement, if you go to a specialist without a GP's referral, insurance will reimburse only 60 percent of the fee; if you have a referral from the GP, insurance repays 70 percent of the bill. For most patients, this means a visit without a referral will cost about $4.50 more. Dr. Tama-let, the orthopedic specialist in Versailles, told me that none of his pa-tients really pays the extra $4.50, because he routinely certifies on the bill that the patient is *parcours coordonné*—that is, "coordinated by" a GP—whether it is true or not.

"OUR HEALTH CARE SYSTEM costs too much," Dr. François Bon-naud told me, "and not enough of the money gets down to the doctor." Dr. Bonnaud, a friendly, dedicated fifty-eight-year-old internist with wire-rim spectacles and bushy black hair, runs a busy family practice. He is also an expert on the French health care system and an officer of the Union Régionale des Médecins Libéraux, the regional union of general practitioners that negotiates with the Health Ministry each year over how much doctors will be paid for medical procedures. I asked Dr. Bonnaud, in his capacity as an expert on the system, why French health care produces better results than the American system for less money. He responded, in his capacity as a family doctor, by inviting me to spend some time in his *cabinet médicale* in the town of Maule so that I could watch French medicine at work. Maule, a town of six thousand about twenty-seven miles west of the Eiffel Tower, is just starting to become a bedroom community for Paris commuters. But it has most of the standard elements of French country villages: an ancient Roman cemetery, a sixteenth-century church with a hand-some rectangular stone steeple, and a market center with a *boulangerie,* a *fromagerie,* and a branch of the farm bank Crédit Agricole. Behind an old stone wall just off the town center is a simple five-room cottage that serves as the clinic for Dr. Bonnaud; his wife, Hélène, another family practitioner, whom he met in medical school; and their partner, Dr. Patrick Chevallier. Their practice has about three thousand patients on its active roster, and the three physicians treat from 70 to 130 pa-tients each day—in the office, in hospitals, and on house calls.

Dr. Bonnaud's crowded, uncarpeted office is about as plain as the chambers of Dr. Tamalet, the orthopedist in Versailles. But Bonnaud's place has some decoration: on one wall, a print of a Matisse still life; on another, a collage of drawings and construction-paper cutouts by his youngest patients. There's an examining table, an eye chart on the wall, a light box for reading X-rays, a small chest that holds bandages and sutures, and the doctor's wooden desk. As in Dr. Tamalet's office, though, something essential seemed to be missing. In the whole building, there was no file cabinet to store the patients' medical records. This conspicuous absence was explained, Dr. Bonnaud told me, by the small green sign on the desk, the same sign I saw at the orthopedist's office and other medical offices throughout France: NOUS ACCEPTONS LA CARTE VITALE.

What that meant became apparent as the day's list of patients began streaming into Dr. Bonnaud's office. At the start of each consultation, the patient handed the doctor a green plastic credit card like this:

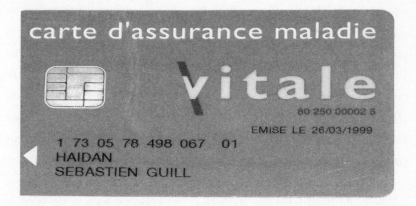

This *carte vitale*—the "vital card," or the "card of life"—contains the patient's entire medical record, back to 1998. Embedded in the gold metallic square just left of center is a digital record of every doctor visit, referral, injection, operation, X-ray, diagnostic test, prescription, warning, etc., together with a report on how much the doctor billed for each visit and how much was paid, by the insurance funds and by the patient. Everybody in France over age fifteen has this card—a child's medical records are maintained on his mother's card—and it is the secret weapon that makes French medical care so much more efficient than anything Americans are used to. When Dr. Bonnaud receives the *carte vitale* from his patient, he slides it into a small reader on top of his desk—it's about the size of a desktop telephone—and the patient's medical record is displayed on the doctor's computer screen. That's why French doctors and hospitals don't need to maintain file cabinets full of records. It's all digitized. It's all on the card. As Dr. Bonnaud considers his patient's symptoms and proposes a remedy—a shot, a course of drugs, a referral to a specialist, a good night's sleep, whatever—he types in a record of the visit and his treatment. That information is written to the patient's *carte vitale*. If the patient is advised to go to the hospital or a specialist or a drugstore, he will take his *carte vitale* along with him, and on it the doctors there will find Dr. Bonnaud's diagnosis and recommended treatment. (With 50 million green cards floating around, a thousand or more get lost every week somewhere in France. If you find a lost card, you're supposed to drop it in any mailbox, and it will be forwarded to the national Centre des Cartes Vitale Perdues, in Le Mans. The Centre says about 80 percent of lost cards eventually get back to the owner.) Because the medical information on that gold chip is encrypted, France's Health Ministry insists that there have been no breaches of patient privacy.

But the greatest value of the *carte vitale* is its impact on the payment of medical bills. Each patient's green card knows which sickness fund and which private health insurance plan (*mutuelle*) covers that patient. When Dr. Bonnaud finishes a consultation and enters that day's treatment on the patient's card, he stretches out the ring finger on his left hand and hits the "transmit" key on his computer. With that single keystroke, all billing information—how much the patient owed, how much he paid the doctor as a co-pay, how much each of the insurance plans should pay back to the doctor and the patient—is transmitted to each of the relevant insurance plans. With that single keystroke, the billing process is finished. "I will be paid," Dr. Bonnaud told me, with total confidence, "in three days." The insurance funds are required to pay him that fast, with no quibbles—and they do.

In addition to the certainty of the process and the resulting peace of mind, this national billing system creates major financial savings. No French doctor, hospital, or drugstore has to pay a "denial management" company to collect what is owed by the health insurance industry. The expensive layer of administrative workers and paper handlers found in every corner of American medicine doesn't exist in France. Dr. Bonnaud told me that he and his partners would never consider hiring a secretary or office manager. "Why would I pay somebody to do my billing?" the doctor said. *"C'est automatique."* Automatic payment also makes French hospitals, public and private, dramatically cheaper to run than any U.S. hospital. Although French hospitals generally have more doctors and nurses per patient than an American establishment, they have 67 percent fewer administrative personnel to keep track of paperwork and billing. "This difference in hospital staffing . . . reflects the difference between a National Health Insurance system and the U.S. health system, characterized by large numbers of administrative and clerical personnel whose main tasks focus on billing many hundreds of payers, documenting all medical procedures performed, and handling risk management and quality assurance activities," notes Professor Victor G. Rodwin, a health policy expert at New York University.[8]

Even though the record-keeping is digital and the billing process is automated, a lot of money changes hands in Dr. Bonnaud's office. The French system expects almost every patient to pay something almost every time he has medical treatment. Most French patients, in fact, pay the full charge for their treatment at the point of service. In Dr. Bonnaud's case, that means cash, plopped down on the doctor's wooden desk once the visit is ended and he has returned the patient's green card. That's why French doctors have such detailed lists of charges, down to the penny, posted in their waiting rooms. For most general practitioners, the basic fee for a consultation with a general practitioner or a family doctor in 2007 was set at 21, or $27.30; for a specialist, the standard rate was 26, or $33.80. These fees tend to go up somewhat every year or so, depending on how noisily the doctors demonstrate during their strikes. But the list of negotiated prices covers everything. Most injections cost about $15, on top of the basic consultation charge. If a patient has a serious cut, Dr. Bonnaud will receive $70 for putting in stitches. Setting a broken arm (evidently considered a simpler process) earns him $61.10; freezing and removing a mole is worth $26.49. To encourage doctors to make house calls, a GP gets an extra $13 for a consultation at the patient's home, and Dr. Bonnaud does a lot of that. When he visits a patient outside the office, he takes along a portable reader for the *carte vitale* and enters all the treatment information onto the card using his laptop computer.

Not quite everybody has to pay in full at the time of treatment. People living below the poverty line and receiving welfare payments are billed just $7.80 for a doctor's visit. The poorest of the poor pay nothing. Anybody certified to be suffering from a chronic illness (*affection de longue durée*) is exempt from payment as well. In those cases, the doctor receives his prescribed fee from the government's social security system. A pregnant woman is exempted from any payment in the last five months of her pregnancy and the first four months after delivery. To limit the cost burden on any individual, the rules say that no patient has to pay more than about $100 in a single day, no matter how much treatment she receives. Aside from those special cases, the French must pay out of pocket every time they see a doctor, go to the hospital, or fill a prescription.

Why? Since the insurance funds will subsequently reimburse the patient for most, or often all, of the cost of medical care, why bother collecting the co-pay across the doctor's desk each time? "Does it seem impractical?" Dr. Bonnaud responded when I asked him. "No, I think it is entirely reasonable. Medical care is a valuable commodity. Its value can be life or death. When we ask the patient to pay that 21 in my office, we remind her that she is receiving a costly service. Even though she's going to get the money back from insurance in a week, maybe two, it is important to convey that something of value is exchanged when they come to see me. And maybe, if somebody calls me to their home just out of loneliness, just to have a chat, maybe that person will spare me the trip because he doesn't want to pay the 31."

Regardless of who pays, the prices for French medicine tend to be seriously cheap. It's hard to imagine any private general practitioner in the United States charging just $27 for an office visit, or any specialist willing to settle for $34 for a normal consultation. Most of the fixed prices set by the Health Ministry amount to one-third, or sometimes one-quarter, of what the same treatment would cost in the United States. Not surprisingly, the cut-rate prices are reflected in doctors' cut-rate incomes. Dr. Bonnaud said he works about sixty hours per week (although he does take the standard five weeks of vacation per year), and his net income, after office expenses, has been about 40,000 ($52,000) per annum in recent years. (He then admitted, with a blush, that the earnings figure is actually a little higher than that, since he bills his Audi to the medical office, even when he uses the car for personal trips.) That's roughly the average income for French general practitioners. Even with the value of the Audi added in, the average French doctor is making about a third of what his counterpart in the United States would earn. Roughly the same income gap applies to French specialists. Dr. Tamalet, my orthopedist, told me that he makes about 50,000 ($65,000) annually as an employee in a government-run hospital, and then earns about the same amount working privately in that spartan office in Versailles. With a combined income of $130,000, he stands far behind the average annual earnings of American shoulder surgeons.

Of course, there are offsetting fiscal considerations. No French doctor pays a penny to go to college or medical school, so none graduates with the kind of debt burden facing most newly minted American M.D.s. In France, as in most of Europe, that's a cost the government bears. French physicians pay less in a year for malpractice insurance—Bonnaud, the GP, pays $170 per year, and Tamalet, the orthopod, pays about $650—than their U.S. counterparts pay in a week. And neither French doctor ever expects to be sued. Even with those benefits, though, French physicans are doing their jobs for far less money than they could make doing the same work in the United States. And they know it.

"I will never be rich," Dr. Bonnaud told me, sitting at the simple wooden desk in his cluttered office. "In the States, I would make much, much more. But there I would be fighting always the insurance companies over what I can prescribe, what I can do for my patients. Here, we have freedom to do the medicine we think is right. And the patient, any patient, can get the treatment needed; the insurance, or the social security, will pay for it. I will never be rich, but I can look in the mirror in the morning and know that I am doing the best for my patients. For a physician, that is a form of richness; it brings satisfaction."

Sometimes, doing the best for his patients means referring them to a specialist for further care. When Dr. Bonnaud saw my stiff, aching shoulder, he did just that: He sent me to Dr. Tamalet in Versailles. After Dr. Tamalet gave me that lecture on France's glorious history of shoulder surgery, he took a close look at my X-rays. He questioned me carefully about the history of my shoulder problem, going back to the initial accident decades earlier. He manipulated my arm and shoulder to get a personal feel for the degree of damage within. And then he delivered his verdict: The smartest thing I could do, he concluded, would be a vigorous regime of physical therapy, to stretch and strengthen the muscular system in my shoulder. That would not eliminate all pain or restore full movement, but it would give me a freer, less painful joint without the risks of major surgery.

I told Dr. Tamalet that my American doctors had proposed a "total shoulder arthroplasty," the modern variant on Dr. Péan's historic intervention in 1892. "Yes, of course, I thought of that," the doctor said, but he decided that I was not a good candidate for a total shoulder replacement. Most of the patients who benefited from that procedure, he said, had different kinds of injuries than I have, and most of them were suffering from constant pain, unlike me. "My recommendation would be that it's not the indicated procedure in your case," the doctor said. But then he pointed out, a little ruefully, that I didn't have to settle for that diagnosis if I didn't like it. "In France, patients have complete freedom of choice—of doctors, of hospitals, of procedures," he said. "You are free to go to any orthopedist. And you would have no trouble finding an orthopedist who would do a total arthroplasty for you. Some surgeon could get 5,000 for doing that operation, and the hospital would keep you for five days, at about 1,000 per day. And the sickness funds would pay for it." I might have to wait a while to get the procedure scheduled at a hospital, the doctor said, but the delay would be no more than a month or so. That's about how long it takes to schedule major surgery in many American cities. "Believe me," Dr. Tamalet summed up, "if you wanted that operation in France, you could get it."

Which is, of course, the boon and the bane of France's health care system. It offers a maximum of free choice among skillful doctors and well-equipped hospitals, with little or no waiting, at bargain-basement prices. It's a system that enables the French to live longer and healthier lives, with zero risk of financial loss due to illness. But somebody has to pay for all that high-quality, ready-when-you-need-it care—and the patients, so far, have not been willing to do so. As a result, the major health insurance funds are all operating at a deficit, and the costs of the health care system are increasing significantly faster than the economy as a whole. That's why the doctors keep striking and the sickness funds keep negotiating and the government keeps going back to the drawing board, with a new "major health care reform" every few years. So far, the saving grace for France's system has been the high level of efficiency, as exemplified by the *carte vitale,* that keeps administrative costs low—much lower than in the United States.

Whatever the next wave of reform might bring, it seems certain that the French will continue to emphasize equal access to medical care—the basic rule that anybody, regardless of race, income, or occupation, can go to any doctor and get the same treatment as anybody else. Whenever the French talk about health care, they invoke the concept of *solidarité,* the notion that all French citizens must stick solidly together to help one another in time of need. "The solidarity principle," explains Professor Rodwin, "requires mutual aid and cooperation among the sick and the well, the inactive and the active, the poor and the wealthy, and insists on financing health insurance on the basis of ability to pay, not actuarial risk."[9]

A French physician, Dr. Valerie Biousse, put the same idea a little more bluntly when I asked her why the French system is so focused on free access to any doctor or hospital. "It would be stupid to say that everybody is equal," she began. "Some are rich and some are poor. Some are beautiful, some aren't. Some are brilliant, some aren't. But when we get sick—then, everybody is equal. Everybody must have equal right to the best medical treatment we can provide." Now Dr. Newman was excited as she rose to her rhetorical climax. "That is the basic rule of French health care," she said. "Surely, that's the basic rule of health care in every country."

Well, not quite. Equal access for all is the basic rule of health care in *almost* every developed country—but not in the United States. But it's not surprising that a European doctor would think this was a universal rule, because the basic idea of a national system providing health care for everybody was a European invention. The notion that government has to create a mechanism to provide medical care for all who are sick was born in the late nineteenth century in the very heart of Europe, in a newly created nation called Germany.

FIVE

Germany: "Applied Christianity"

AMID A TOWERING GROVE OF MAPLES NEAR THE CENTER OF the Tiergarten, Berlin's equivalent of Central Park, stands the Bismarck Memorial, a colossal bronze statue, much larger than life, that depicts a nineteenth-century hero in a field marshal's uniform, with a saber in his hand, a spiked helmet on his head, and a look of ferocious determination beneath his furrowed brow. The whole aspect suggests a ruthless hunger for power, and in that sense the elaborate monument is an accurate depiction of Otto von Bismarck, the "Iron Chancellor" who unified the German nation to create an industrial and military powerhouse at the center of Europe. When he set out, in 1862, to fuse a dozen fiefdoms and principalities into a single German *Reich*, Bismarck warned that the task would be achieved "not by speeches and the resolutions of majorities, but by iron and blood." The chancellor dominated his German Empire for three decades largely by iron and blood, never hindered by abstractions like democracy or the rule of law if they stood in the way of personal or national ambition.

And thus it is somewhat counterintuitive to think of Bismarck as a humanitarian leader who wanted to help ordinary people deal with hardships like sickness and accidents. In fact, though, the Iron Chancellor had a benevolent streak. Always an innovator, Bismarck originated several of the programs that make up the modern welfare state. (As we'll see shortly, historians are still trying to figure out what prompted him to do it.) His Sickness Insurance Law, enacted by the Reichstag in 1883, was the world's first national health care system. It was a program of mandatory medical insurance, with premiums paid jointly by employees and workers. For ease of administration, the worker's share was withheld automatically from his pay. To this day, the 1883 structure remains a model for nations around the world. American workers who buy a health insurance plan through their employer, with the premium withheld from the paycheck, are using the Bismarck Model of health care.

In its home country today, the Bismarck health care system guarantees medical care to just about all 82 million Germans and to millions of "guest workers," legal or not, who live in the country. The package of benefits is generous, covering doctors, dentists, chiropractors, physical therapists, psychiatrists, hospitals, opticians, all prescriptions, nursing homes, health club memberships, and even vacation trips to a spa (when suggested by a doctor). The quality of care is world-class; Germany stands at or near the top in all comparative health care studies. Because the supply of hospitals and doctors is ample, there's no "queue" for treatment; on measures such as "waiting time for emergency care" and "waiting time for elective/non-emergency surgery," Germans spend less time waiting for care than Americans do.[1] Patients can choose any doctor or hospital, and insurance must pay the bill. And every German has a choice among some two hundred different private insurance plans, which compete vigorously even though the prices for insurance are fixed.

It's worth emphasizing that the insurance plans—that is, the *Krankenkassen,* or "sickness funds"—are private entities. The general practitioners who make up the bulk of Germany's medical profession are also private businesspeople, working in private clinics. German hospitals are mainly charity or municipal operations, but there is a growing business in private, for-profit hospital chains. The private insurance plans negotiate prices with the private medical clinics and the hospitals; these are private commercial agreements, with little government input. In many areas of medical practice, there's less government control of medical care in Germany than in the United States. It's sheer nonsense to suggest that Germany, or any of the other countries using the Bismarck approach, is engaged in government-run "socialized medicine."

But there's a downside, of course, and a serious one. Providing free choice of insurance and treatment, in a system with minimal waiting and a high standard of quality, costs money. Germany has one of the world's more expensive health care systems, consuming nearly 11 percent of the nation's hefty GDP. That's significantly higher than in most other European nations. Still, the German system is a bargain-basement operation compared to the United States, where we spend about 17 percent of GDP on a health care system that provides less choice and less coverage than Germany does. To pay for its expensive system, Germany strictly controls payments to doctors and hospitals, and the system is constantly looking for ways to cut spending. Among other things, German health care has far lower administrative costs than the U.S. system. The advent in 2008 of a universal smart card, known as *die elektronischen Gesundheitskarte* ("the digital health card"), has eliminated much paperwork and reduced administrative costs even further. It galls the Germans a little that they were slower than the French in switching to digital records; on the other hand, they made the switch long before the United States was ready to do so, and that mitigates the gloom somewhat.

Because the German system offers such a big benefits package, I was not greatly surprised with the activist German response to my shoulder problem. German doctors were just about as quick as my American orthopedist to suggest the high-priced, no-holds-barred surgical solution: total replacement with a man-made shoulder.

I first took my bum shoulder to Dr. Christina von Köckritz, a slender, talkative mother of four who practices as a *Hausarzt,* or family doctor, in the pleasant lakeside village of Kladow, south of Berlin. Dr. Christina is a serious and extremely hardworking woman, but she is also a person who cares about style. She wears tailored white slacks, a white polo shirt, and a white doctor's coat. She practices in a modern, spotless office furnished with a white desk, white chairs, and a small white sonogram machine; even the oxygen tank on the wall is sleek and white. A Mark Rothko print on the wall, with its big blocks of red and yellow, tends to emphasize the whiteness of everything else in this attractive setting.

In her role as the gatekeeper controlling my access to German health care, Dr. Christina palpated and manipulated my shoulder, studied the X-rays, and then looked up my condition in a detailed online directory called the Gebührenordnung für Ärtze, or GOÄ. This is the crucial document of German health care; the product of extensive negotiations between the sickness funds and the doctors' union, it tells both doctor and patient what procedures and treatments the insurance system will cover. As it turned out, the GOÄ gave a green light in my case to a total shoulder arthroplasty, the shoulder-replacement surgery originally proposed by my doctor back home. For anyone covered by one of the sickness funds—that is, almost any German—the price of this procedure in Germany would come to about $30; that is, a couple of co-payments, one for the doctor's office and one for hospital admission.

Dr. Christina was ready to direct me to an orthopedic surgeon who could examine me and perform the surgery, probably within a week. Still, she urged me to take my time about it, to talk to the surgeon and to a physical therapist before plunging into surgery. Like Dr. Tamalet, the orthopod in Versailles, she felt that a total shoulder replacement was not the best remedy for my type of injury. And yet, if I had chosen to have the operation, the German system would have provided it.

To me, German health care looked good: high quality, easy access without waiting, reasonable costs (for the patient, at least). But as I talked to doctors, patients, and government health officials, I sensed that Germans don't feel the same affection for their system that I found among the French. Physicians, in particular, have been complaining for years about the fees they receive from the sickness funds; the sickness funds and the government, meanwhile, are worried about relentless increases in cost. As a result, new German governments routinely offer programs for "health care reform," and significant changes have been made in the past decade or so. But the basic system remains unchanged. The basic model—private health insurance provided through employers, with government acting as an umpire—has survived 125 years and massive political turmoil. The Bismarck era led to Germany's shattering defeat in World War I, which led to the Weimar Republic (twenty-one governments in fourteen years), which led to the Nazis, which led to Germany's shattering defeat in World War II, which led to the division of the country and the Berlin Wall and eventually to today's united democratic Germany. Through all those political convolutions, the nation has stuck with the health care model designed by Otto von Bismarck.

OTTO EDUARD LEOPOLD VON BISMARCK was born in 1815, six weeks before the battle of Waterloo ended Napoleon's effort to redraw the map of Europe. By the time of his death, eighty-three years later, Bismarck was widely compared to Napoleon, not as a military commander but, rather, as the dominant political and diplomatic force on the Continent. He grew up in a prominent family in Prussia, a kingdom comprising what are now northeast Germany and Poland. He was a quick learner—he mastered Greek, Latin, French, English, and Russian while in school—but not exactly a diligent student. As an undergraduate at the great university in Göttingen, "he spent his time womanizing, fighting duels, playing roulette and drinking his companions under the table."[2] All his life, he had a fiery temper; when a would-be assassin with a handgun approached him and started firing in 1866, Bismarck was so outraged that he stepped past his bodyguards, grabbed the assailant by the neck, and wrenched him violently to the ground. (Fortunately, the gunman was a rotten shot.) He loved food and drink, and it showed. Bismarck was not only the first German chancellor but also the fattest.

Taking advantage of family connections, Bismarck served in the Prussian legislature and later became one of the kingdom's top diplomats. The fateful moment of his career came in 1862, when he was Prussia's ambassador in Paris. The kaiser summoned him home to become "minister-president"—in effect, prime minister—of Prussia. Bismarck also assumed the post of foreign minister, recognizing that his main tasks would be dealing with other major European powers and with the numerous German-speaking states that were then joined in a loose customs union. Using the mighty Prussian army as his instrument, Bismarck launched a series of wars and annexations that collected most of the independent Germanic states into the nation of Germany. In January of 1871, he formally declared the birth of the Deutsches Reich, or German Empire, a new nation that included all of today's Germany, plus large swatches that are now part of France, Denmark, and Poland. The national capital, naturally, was set in the old Prussian capital, Berlin. With this great work completed, the minister-president of Prussia became the chancellor of Germany. But he did not demur when underlings addressed him by the more ornate title *Reichsgründer,* "Founder of the Nation."

For two decades, the Iron Chancellor fought bitter political battles against competing parties, striving to keep the new country united and his personal power intact. His primary adversaries were the Catholic Church, which he viewed as a reactionary force on the right, and the rising Socialist Party, fighting his policies from the left. Toward the opposition, Bismarck was not gentle. He deported priests, jailed political enemies, and shut down opposition newspapers; he rejected almost any policy idea that was not his own. He hated taxes; at one point, he threatened to move out of Berlin, taking the national government with him, if the city didn't reduce the property tax on his own house. Accordingly, he struggled to minimize public spending; he tried (in vain) to finance the whole government with the income from import duties.

As head of this new nation, Bismarck saw that his historic role would be to create Germany not simply as a legal entity but as a political, financial, and cultural union. One way to do that was to provide benefits for people in every region of the *Reich*—to give Bavarians, Hanoverians, Frankfurters, and everyone else a sense of belonging, of gratitude, toward the new national government in Berlin. And thus Bismarck invented the welfare state. He pushed through an "Accident Insurance Law"—in modern parlance, a workmen's-compensation system—to provide medical treatment and financial payments for workers hurt on the job. He created an old-age pension system—a social security system. And he authored the Sickness Insurance Law of 1883, to assure that any injured or ailing German could obtain medical treatment. To keep taxes low, Bismarck financed much of his welfare program through private insurance plans. He built his health care system around an existing network of sickness funds, run on a nonprofit basis by industrial guilds and unions. Under the 1883 law, each employee had to join and pay into one of the sickness funds, with the employer chipping in to help pay the premium. The result was a national health care system that didn't require any tax revenues. In its original manifestation, the new system paid all the medical bills of covered workers and their families. For the first time in history, a government created a mechanism to ensure that any citizen, rich or poor, could obtain medical treatment for illness or injury.

For the past century or so, historians have been debating why a crotchety, tax-averse, right-wing aristocrat like Bismarck would invest so much of his political capital in welfare benefits for the working class. Some of the explanations involve practical politics: Bismarck's new national government needed to win the allegiance of the entire German population, and a welfare state helped do that. He needed a healthy workforce to man the factories of a rapidly industrializing modern economy. He needed healthy young men to form a German army and navy. He needed to offer welfare benefits as a pacifier for a populace that had almost no role in government—"He introduced social rights to avoid granting wider political rights," as the historian Paul Starr put it.[3] As a cunning politician, the chancellor needed programs that would undermine political support for the Socialists and other left-wing parties. To do that, he appropriated their policies and made them his own—just as a liberal Democratic president of the United States pushed for welfare reform, and a conservative Republican president added prescription-drug benefits to Medicare. Indeed, Bismarck even appropriated his opponents' language, calling his welfare program *Der Staatssozialismus,* or "state socialism."

Beyond all those pragmatic explanations, though, it seems that Otto von Bismarck was driven as well by a charitable impulse, perhaps a product of his Lutheran upbringing. When the chancellor first proposed his welfare state to the Reichstag, in 1881, he described it as a means for the more fortunate Germans to care for the least of their brethren; public welfare, he said, should be viewed as "a program of applied Christianity." Defending his medical and unemployment insurance schemes in 1884, Bismarck argued that "the greatest burden for the working class is the uncertainty of life. They can never be certain that they will have a job, or that they will have health and the ability to work. We cannot protect a man from all sickness and misfortune.

But it is our obligation, as a society, to provide assistance when he encounters these difficulties. . . . A rich society must care for the poor."[4]

The Iron Chancellor ruled with an iron hand for three decades. By the end of the 1880s, though, it was clear that his passion for power was fading. He stayed mainly at his country manor, rarely making an appearance in the capital. He grew fatter than ever. In the parliamentary election of 1890, his conservative coalition was driven from power. After twenty-five years as the first statesman of Europe, Bismarck retreated to his wheelchair and his memories; he died in 1898. He may have foreseen the terrible upheaval that his German Empire would endure in the twentieth century. He told a colleague that all his military and diplomatic triumphs might "come to nothing" in the new century. But some aspects of his work would endure, he predicted: "The programs of state socialism will dig themselves in."[5]

AS THAT FIRST Sickness Insurance Law of 1883 contemplated, Germans today are required to belong to a sickness fund. At the beginning of the twenty-first century there were about four hundred of these *Krankenkassen,* but a wave of mergers is reducing the number; in mid-2010, there were about 180 insurance funds. On a regional basis, they negotiate pricing arrangements with hospitals and doctors' associations. The price established in this agreement becomes the fixed price for all physicians and hospitals in the region. For the patient, this price is basically irrelevant; the doctor collects her fee from the sickness fund, and the patient never sees a bill. The patient pays a monthly insurance premium to the fund; this fee is a percentage of income (like the Social Security tax in the United States), so that high earners pay more for the same coverage. As the cost of medicine has risen, the insurance premium has risen as well. Currently, Germans pay about 15 percent of their paycheck for health insurance, split between the worker and the employer. That's almost exactly equal to what an American worker and his employer pay in Social Security and Medicare taxes. But the German worker gets a better deal. Most American workers also have to pay a health insurance premium, ranging from 2 to 10 percent of pay, in addition to those payroll taxes.

A private health insurance plan, funded by payroll withholding, that pays doctors and hospitals directly on a fee-for-service basis—that's the classic Bismarck Model, and it sounds very much like American-style employer-based medical insurance. But the German version of Bismarck is different in three fundamental ways:

1. First and foremost, the sickness funds are nonprofit entities; they exist to pay people's medical bills, not to pay dividends to shareholders. Thus, they don't have the same incentive that the U.S. insurance industry has to limit the people they cover or to deny claims; in fact, the German insurance plans are required to accept all applicants and to pay any claims submitted by a recognized doctor or hospital. They don't have to pad their premiums to pay for a claims-review bureaucracy or to allow for profit. The result: The sickness funds have about one-third the administrative expenses that are normal in American health insurance. That makes the whole German insurance system much cheaper.

2. While insurance is purchased and paid for through payroll deduction, Germans don't lose their coverage when they lose their jobs. Government unemployment benefits automatically cover the insurance premium, so the worker has the same insurance coverage while he looks for a new job—no matter how long it takes to find one.

3. Unlike American workers, who are restricted to the limited selection of insurance plans offered by their employers, Ger-

mans can sign up with any sickness fund in the country and can change to a different plan almost anytime they want. To a large extent, the funds all mimic one another. They are all required by law to offer the mandated package of benefits, from cradle to nursing home. Since the premium is a percentage of pay, the premium stays the same, no matter which fund a worker chooses. And yet there is heated competition among these nonprofit insurance plans. Some compete by promising to pay all claims within five days; some offer benefits beyond the basic package, like exotic Asian therapies or free neonatal nursing care in the home after a baby is born or longer stays in those health spas.

Among health care economists, the consumer's free choice of any insurance plan, and the resulting competition among the insurers, is one of the most admired features of the German system. "Americans tend to think that the profit motive is the only driver of competition," Karl Lauterbach, a German economist who won a seat in the Bundestag, the national parliament, told me. "But our *Krankenkassen* compete because the executives earn more money, and higher prestige, if they have a larger pool of insured members. So we have universal coverage, and nobody can be turned down because of a preexisting illness. You have the required package of benefits, so the insurer can't deny a claim for any covered treatment. And then you have this competition to attract more customers."

The sickness funds cover almost all Germans, but not everybody. Following a principle established in Bismarck's original plan, the richest families are excused from the mandated insurance, on the theory that they don't need help getting health care. Those who don't join a sickness fund can buy private coverage from profit-making insurance firms; about 7 percent of the population chooses this option. Some private hospitals cater to this segment, offering more luxurious facilities and famous doctors; these institutions charge higher prices than the sickness funds would pay. This is controversial. Liberal parties complain that this waiver for the wealthy undermines the principle of national solidarity; conservatives say it provides a useful relief valve for the basic system. Since the mandatory system is already-facing stiff budget problems, it seems unlikely that the 7 percent of Germans who choose to stay outside it will be brought into it anytime soon.

Like every health care system on earth, Germany's has been heavily influenced in recent decades by advances in treatment and medication, and the big increase in costs resulting from these expensive technologies. The government and the sickness funds have responded with a series of cost-control measures and incentives to reduce the burdens on the system. For patients, the most controversial change happened on January 1, 2006; from that day forth, German patients were required to make a cash payment when they visited a doctor's office or hospital. By global standards, this co-pay is tiny: You have to come up with 10—that is, $13 or so—each quarter of the year. Once you've paid the $13, all services are free for the rest of the quarter. Still, Germans were outraged—a visit to the doctor should be free, everyone knew that. Americans living in Germany took this small fee in stride. Dr. Christina told me that many American expatriates live in her town, and several are her patients. One came in to see her in January of 2006. Christina told him, apologetically, that the rules had just changed; from now on, he would have to pay 10 in cash to see the doctor. The American patient paid without complaint. Ten weeks later, in the middle of March, the same patient came back for another consultation. "And the funny thing is," Christina said with a laugh, "he reached in his pocket and tried to pay me 10 again—twice in the same quarter!" Clearly, the doctor found this amusing. "What happens in America?" she asked me. "Do people expect to make a payment every time they go to a doctor's office?"

ON A COLD, WET, and generally miserable March day, the famous Berlin avenue Unter den Linden ("under the linden trees") was swarming with angry men and women, many wearing white doctors' coats. Tens of thousands of physicians, nurses, and medical students had turned out for a noisy demonstration against the latest round of health care reform proposals endorsed by the government of Chancellor Angela Merkel. In the midst of that mob, wearing tailored white slacks, a white shirt, a white doctor's coat, and a stethoscope around her neck, stood Christina von Köckritz, the family doctor who was my guide to German medicine. Dr. Christina told me later that she was uncomfortable in that noisy demonstration. She was cold. She was wet. And she was seriously conflicted as to whether a physician rightly ought to be marching down the street toward the Reichstag chanting antigovernment catcalls.

"I think, yes, a doctor would rather be in the clinic, to make medicine," she told me in her clear but somewhat rusty English. "I think about twenty thousand doctors, to demonstrate in the street, that is not usual. But the situation we are in! The budgets, and too much papers, too much bureaucracy. So we did demo, we did march, hoping that we could take better care of our patients without all the changes. But it mattered nothing. The government is changing medicine, and now we cannot make good medicine so much as we used to."

But there are offsetting considerations. As is common in Europe, Christina's medical education was free; she never faced any student debt. For a busy general practice with more than seven hundred active patients, she pays about $1,400 per year for malpractice insurance— barely one week's premium for many American family doctors. In twenty-four years of practice, she has never been sued. Although her patients use many different sickness funds, all the plans follow the same rules and the same payment formula, which is set forth clearly in the

GOÄ directory. Other than the newly instituted co-pay, she never has to bill or collect from a patient. The insurance plans pay her within a week or so; she has never had a claim denied.

Why, then, have the streets of Berlin been filled with angry doctors protesting the health care system? The reason is that Germany, like most developed countries, finds it difficult to control the accelerating costs of medical care. The most common cost-control methodology for the sickness funds and for the Merkel government has been to target the medical profession. A series of "reforms" over the past decade or so has led to tough new controls over the treatments doctors can choose, the medications they can prescribe, and the money they can earn. Those are the changes that drew the mild-mannered physician Christina von Köckritz, somewhat to her own surprise, to join the white-coated legions on the Unter den Linden that cold March morning in 2006.

Dr. Christina became a widow in the mid-1990s, when the youngest of her four children was still an infant. In the years since, she has struggled, sometimes to the point of exhaustion, to balance her solo medical practice in Kladow with the demands of raising and supporting her family. "I am a mother," she told me plaintively. "I can't be at the office twelve hours per day." She sees dozens of patients in her examining room each day, and most weeks she sets aside two half days for house calls on patients who are bedridden. After she pays her four employees and the other expenses of her office, she earns somewhere between $100,000 and $150,000 per year. It's a decent income—although she notes with a touch of bitterness that an American doctor with a similar practice in most U.S. cities would make significantly more for the same work. The real problem is that recent health care reforms in Germany are beginning to reduce her pay.

To get control over costs, the German Health Ministry has authorized the sickness funds to use a system known as "global budgeting." In essence, this means that the health system agrees to spend a certain amount of money each year—and stops paying for care when that budget is reached. Global budgeting is fairly common in health care systems with strong central controls—the Beveridge Model systems, like Britain's National Health Service and the U.S. Department of Veterans Affairs, have used it for years—but it was unknown in Germany until the reforms of 2002. Now the sickness funds in Christina's region are trying to put an absolute lid on expenditures for treatment. In her case, the insurance system pays her to see about seven hundred different patients per quarter. Although there are some mechanisms to get around the limit, this means essentially that she won't be paid for treating the 701st patient who walks in the door. "I theoretically, I could stop after that point," she told me, "and go on vacation for three weeks. Many doctors do, yes? But you don't do it as a family doctor. If the patients [are] sick, you must treat. For that patient, you must be a doctor for no pay until the next quarter."

To make up for the lost income, Dr. Christina has become an entrepreneur. She now offers a broad range of treatments and classes in cosmetic medicine, hair removal, liposuction, exercise techniques, etc., aimed primarily at working women like herself. A plaque on the white wall of the waiting room notes that Dr. Von Köckritz has obtained a Zertifikat am Intensivkurs Botulinumtoxin, which means she can offer Botox injections. She has installed an exercise machine—basically, a fancy treadmill—and she charges customers about $15 per half hour to use it. None of these services is covered by the basic health insurance plan—and that's the beauty of them for Dr. Christina. She sets the fees herself for these treatments, receiving payment directly from the patients, and that income doesn't count against the system's "global budget." "I must learn new things, a lot, to make money," the doctor told me. "It is not what I thought I would do when I was in medical school. I cannot say I like it. But this is German medicine practice today."

———

To an American visiting the country on a quest for a cure, German medicine practice today looks good. On a personal level, the German system was ready to handle my shoulder problem. Had I been a member of any sickness fund, I could have chosen to have the surgical solution, total shoulder arthroplasty, at a rock-bottom price, with no waiting. If that approach seemed too drastic, the German insurance plans would have paid for less radical remedies, like physical therapy or injections for pain. On a national level, Germany offers universal care through private insurance that is available to everybody. The intense rivalry among the sickness funds demonstrates that there can be elements of the competitive free market even in a nonprofit health insurance system. Patients report high levels of satisfaction—and they should, given the broad range of care they get in return for moderate insurance premiums and a tiny co-pay. And yet, the system is plagued by relentless cost increases. To counter that trend, the sickness funds and the government are squeezing the providers of medical care, the physicians and the hospitals. And the doctors, in turn, are marching in the streets.

The health care system that Otto von Bismarck created still works. But even after 125 years of German engineering, it is not perfect.

SIX

Japan: Bismarck on Rice

DURING A DEBATE AMONG THE PRESIDENTIAL CANDIDATES in the spring of 2008, former New York mayor Rudy Giuliani offered a picture of health care in foreign countries: "These countries that say they provide universal coverage—they pay a price for it, you know," Giuliani explained. "They do it by rationing care, by long waiting lines, and by limiting, or I should say by eliminating, a patient's choice." Judging from that, it seems safe to say that Rudy Giuliani has never visited Dr. Nakamichi Noriaki at the Orthopedic Surgery Department of Keio Daigaku Hospital in Tokyo.

In a society that is acutely conscious of hierarchy and rank, Dr. Nakamichi is generally recognized as one of the top orthopedic surgeons in all Japan; his clinic at Keio is perhaps the most respected place in the country for the repair of stiff, aching shoulders like mine. I was first told about him one Thursday morning in Tokyo when I was complaining, as usual, about my shoulder. I called his office to schedule an appointment—and was told to come in that same afternoon. After the familiar poking, patting, massage, and manipulation, Dr. Nakamichi suggested an assortment of different treatments that might work for me; in fact, it was the widest variety of care any doctor had proposed. The treatment available in Japan ranges from acupuncture to injections to manipulation to the total shoulder arthroplasty that my doctor back home had recommended. All the options, he told me, are covered by Japanese health insurance. When I asked how long I would have to wait if I chose the full-scale shoulder-replacement surgery, the doctor checked his computer. "Tomorrow would be a little difficult," he said. "But next week would probably work."

In other words: no waiting, no gatekeeper, no rationing, and a broad array of patient choice. Prices are low; as we'll see, the Japanese system has a rigid cost-control mechanism that favors the patient, at the expense of doctors and hospitals. My out-of-pocket cost for an office visit with the prestigious Dr. Nakamichi in his prestigious clinic came to ¥2,060, or $19 (the doctor charged $64, and insurance pays 70 percent of the bill in Japan). Had I chosen to have the shoulder-replacement surgery in Tokyo, the total price—including five nights in the hospital—would have run about $10,000. That's roughly one-fourth of what the operation would cost in the USA, assuming one night in the hospital.

It's worth noting that this happens in a largely private-sector system; Japan relies on private doctors and hospitals, with the bills paid by insurance plans. In fact, Japanese doctors are the most capitalist, and most competitive, that I've seen anywhere in the world. Japanese clinics and hospitals blanket the buses, the subways, the billboards, and the airwaves with advertising. A Tokyo doctor named Yamamoto Hidehiro advertises that he can solve the problem of chronically sweaty palms—evidently, this is a problem in Japan. His Yamamoto Clinic places ads on the commuter trains with disgusting pictures of sweat-drenched hands that his methods have cured. (If you want to see this stuff, you can check his Web site, www.tenoase.com, which is Japanese for "www.sweatyhands. com.") Another Tokyo doctor calls himself Dr. Kuro and specializes in the regrowth of hair on balding scalps. He runs TV commercials that show a group of comely nurses in extremely short white uniforms who sing the clinic's telephone number. It is 09-696-9696. In Japanese, the combination 9-6 can be pronounced "ku-ro," so the nurses sing "kuro-kuro-kuro-kuro." As you've probably guessed, *kuro* just happens to be a Japanese word for thick black hair.

Since medical care is so readily available, so easy to get, and so cheap, you might think that the Japanese use an awful lot of medical care. And you'd be right. The Japanese are the world's most prodigious consumers of health care.[1] The average Japanese visits a doctor about 14.5 times per year—three times as often as the U.S. average, and twice as often as any nation in Europe. If you can't get to the doctor, no problem: Nearly all general practitioners in Japan make house calls, either daily or weekly. The Japanese love medical technology; they get twice as many CAT scans per capita as Americans do and three times as many MRI scans. Japan has twice as many hospital beds per capita as the United States, and people use them. The average hospital stay in Japan is thirty-six nights, compared to six nights in the United States. Japanese women giving birth consider it routine to stay in the hospital with their infants for eight to ten days—roughly a week longer than a new mother in the United States. Japan lags, though, in terms of invasive surgery; Japanese patients are much less apt than Americans to have operations such as arthroplasty, transplant, or heart bypass. This is partly economics—since the fees for surgery are low, doctors don't recommend it as often—and partly cultural. As a rule, Japanese doctors and patients prefer drugs to cutting the body. On a per-capita basis, the Japanese take about twice as many prescription drugs as Americans do.

And yet, statistics tell us that the Japanese don't really need to go to the doctor. By many measures, they are the healthiest people on earth. Japan leads the world in life expectancy (85.5 years for women, 78.7 for men) and in the more relevant statistic, healthy life expectancy at age sixty. (This helps explain the low rate of surgery.) The national health statistics suggest that the quality of Japanese medicine is high: Without good doctors, people would presumably succumb to illness and die younger. But quality medical care is not the only reason for Japan's healthy population.

"Japan's macro health indices, such as healthy life expectancy and infant mortality, are the best, or among the best, in the world," says Professor Ikegami Naoki, the country's best-known health care economist. "Now, that's not all the result of health care. Japan has lower rates of violent crime than most countries, less illicit drug use, fewer traffic accidents, lower rates of HIV infection, less obesity. In terms of keeping people alive and healthy, those factors obviously help. But you also have to give some credit to the health care system for providing universal coverage and egalitarian access without long waiting lists, and we need to credit the doctors and the medical schools for providing a high quality of treatment."

The Japanese system, in short, provides care to every resident of Japan, for minimal fees, with no waiting lists—and excellent results. This is a good deal for the people of Japan, and they take advantage of it, flocking to clinics and hospitals. To an American, it seems natural that this formula—heavy demand by an aging population, with almost no rationing of care—would add up to a huge national medical bill. But when it comes to costs, Japan has turned the predictable formula upside down. Despite universal coverage and prodigious consumption, Japan spends a lot less for health care than most of the developed nations; with costs running at about 8 percent of GDP, it spends about half as much as the United States.

Americans consider it inevitable that health care costs always go up, generally increasing faster than the overall rate of inflation. In the United States and most other countries, that's true. Japan has turned that expectation upside down as well. From the mid-1990s into the first years of the twenty-first century, Japanese health care costs held steady and even dropped on a year-to-year basis several times. That was a period of economic doldrums and deflation in Japan. But even in 2006, when the economy was growing again, Japan's total spending on health care decreased by 3.16 percent from the year before.

As we'll see shortly, not everybody in Japan is happy with the system and its strict cost controls, because the system squeezes cost by sharply limiting the income of medical providers—doctors, nurses, hospitals, labs, drug makers. But if your goal is to provide quality care for everybody at a reasonable cost (which is not a bad goal for any health system), then the Japanese model could be a good one to follow.

It's a model familiar to Americans who buy private health insurance through their employers. Health care in Japan is paid for through insurance plans; generally, the patient has to pay 30 percent of the doctor bill as a co-pay, and the insurance company picks up the remaining 70 percent. (The co-pay is lower for children and the elderly.) There's a monthly limit on a patient's payments, however; nobody has to pay more than about $650 in a month. If I had chosen that $10,000 arthroplasty at Keio Daigaku Hospital, it would have cost me roughly $650 out of pocket, and insurance would have paid the remainder of the bill. The insurance plans must accept everyone who applies, regardless of preexisiting conditions, and they must pay every bill submitted by a physician or a hospital. They can't turn you down for coverage, and they can't deny your claim.

At its core, this is the familiar Bismarck Model, with private, albeit nonprofit, insurance plans paying private providers. But the Japanese variation has some distinctive elements. One striking fact about Japan's version of Bismarck is how many different health insurance plans there are. France has 14 plans, serving different professions. Germany has something over 200 sickness funds. But Japan has about 3,500 health insurance plans. They fall into three general categories, with varying degrees of government involvement.[2]

1. The most common are the plans set up by large companies and large government agencies to cover their employees; the premiums are split between employer and employee, with the company required to pay about 55 percent of the cost. These big-employer plans are self-supporting; they get no subsidy from the government. In fact, the big companies are required to pay for most of the health insurance for their own employees and to subsidize the separate insurance plan for pensioners. Many big companies in Japan, including Toyota and Honda, maintain large hospitals for their employees, again with no public subsidy.

2. For people who work in smaller companies, there is a separate tier of insurance plans. For these plans, too, the worker and the employer split the premium, but the small companies get help from the national government, which pays about 14 percent of the insurance costs.

3. Finally, there is the Citizens Health Insurance plan, for retirees and the self-employed. In this plan, the individual and the local government split the cost of the premium.

Everyone in Japan is required to sign up with a health insurance plan. This is what's known as an "individual mandate," a concept that has sparked furious debate in the United States. But every nation that relies on health insurance has that requirement —it's necessary to ensure a viable risk pool for the insurance companies—and in Japan the mandate is not controversial at all. "It's considered an element of personal responsibility, that you insure yourself against health care costs," Dr. Ikegami told me. "And who can be against personal responsibility?"

An individual mandate to buy insurance raises a corollary question: How do you enforce the mandate? That is an issue America's policy makers have debated time and again, with no real resolution. Japan has come up with a fairly elegant solution to this common problem. If you don't have an insurance plan, you'll be assigned to one run by your local city government. If you don't pay the premium—about 1 percent of the population fails to pay—you'll get regular dunning letters from the insurance company. But if you get sick, you're required to pay all the back premiums you have missed (up to one year's worth) before the insurance company will pay your bill. The result is that the few people who refuse to pay health insurance premiums tend to make up their arrears when they have an accident or become seriously ill. For the unemployed, or those too poor to pay their premium, local government pays the insurance premium instead, so coverage never lapses.

It's not a coincidence that the Japanese system of private providers and private, nonprofit insurance companies follows the Bismarck Model. At a pivotal moment in their history, the Japanese looked around the world for ideas on governing a modern nation. When it came to social welfare, including health care, they decided to copy the system set up in Germany by Otto von Bismarck.

UNTIL THE SECOND HALF of the nineteenth century, Japan was a feudal agricultural society; the island nation had deliberately cut itself off from the rest of the world. Japan in 1850 had an emperor in a lavish palace who was actually a figurehead with no power to govern. A military family, the Tokugawa, ruled the country through a collection of regional warlords who had to answer, in turn, to a dictator called the shogun. For 250 years, the Tokugawa shoguns held to a policy of strict isolation from other countries. On a few occasions, Japanese fishermen were shipwrecked and plucked from the sea by foreign ships; when these unfortunates were returned to Japan, the shogun immediately had them beheaded lest they taint the population with alien ideas.

This enforced isolationism evaporated virtually overnight. In 1853,

Commodore Matthew Perry sailed into Tokyo Bay with a U.S. Navy squadron of coal-fired ships—a technological development Japan had never seen before. Quickly recognizing that samurai swords and the ancient warrior code could not stand up to this modern, mechanized fleet and its powerful cannons, the Japanese submitted. The shogun was overthrown. A reform-minded group of leaders took control, acting, in standard Japanese fashion, in the name of a figurehead ruler, the emperor Meiji. The Meiji reformers set out to turn backward Japan into a modern, industrialized nation. To do that, they sent teams of bright young men, many of them former samurai, to the United States and Europe to learn how modern nations worked. These study teams borrowed the best ideas they found in each country and brought them home. Over three decades, Japan created a military modeled on the German army and a seafaring force copied from the British navy. They instituted France's Code Napoléon as a legal system. They brought in Brits to build railroads and Americans to string telegraph lines. They built German-style elementary and middle schools, complete with militaristic uniforms, and universities based on Oxford and Cambridge, complete with top hats for the students. A former samurai, Iwasaki Yataro, hired Dutch naval engineers to build a shipping company; he named his new enterprise after the design on the Iwasaki family crest: "Three Diamonds" or "Mitsubishi." Impressed by the vast farms of the American Midwest, the reformers started a dairy industry in the vast, empty northern island of Hokkaido; to this day, a visitor there will run across herds, pastures, silos, and red-roofed barns that look like rural Wisconsin.

In terms of social welfare, the world's leading model of modernization at the time of the Meiji reforms was Bismarck's Germany. The Japanese saw and admired the chancellor's network of health and accident insurance plans designed to unify the country and keep the workforce healthy. The Japanese brought German doctors and economists to the newly established University of Tokyo to teach the nation how to practice, and manage, Western medicine. Japan adopted the Bismarck Model: Workers obtained health insurance through the employer, and the premium was split between the employee and the company. Because most of the Japanese workforce was employed on farms or in small family businesses, the government also created a separate network of insurance plans to cover people not working in big companies. The third insurance network, for the elderly and the self-employed, was established after World War II.

As in other nations (except the United States) that use the Bismarck Model, Japanese health insurance companies are nonprofit; they exist to pay medical bills, not to earn a profit for investors. As in Germany, a worker who loses his job keeps his health insurance, with government picking up the employer's share of the premium. But Japanese health care differs from the German system in some important ways:

- The Japanese require that everybody buy insurance (the Germans excuse people in the highest income bracket from this mandate).

- Germany lets any citizen buy into any of the country's two hundred sickness funds; in Japan, there is no choice of insurance plan. You have to get your insurance from your employer (or your spouse/parent's employer) or the local municipality. Japanese patients have freedom in picking a doctor or hospital, but no freedom to choose among insurance plans.

- In Germany, the insurance plans negotiate prices with doctors and hospitals on a regional basis. In Japan, the government—specifically, the Ministry of Health and Welfare—does the negotiating with providers. The result of this negotiation is a single Fee Schedule that applies to every doctor, clinic, and hospital in Japan, from the priciest Tokyo suburbs to remote islands off the coast of rural prefectures. And that Fee

Schedule helps explain one more major difference between
Japan and Germany:

- Germany has one of the more expensive health care systems
  in the developed world, accounting for nearly 11 percent of
  GDP—and costs are rising. Japan, with the same universal
  coverage as Germany and results that are at least as good,
  spends only 8 percent of GDP on health care, with little or
  no increase in costs from year to year.

The tight cost control, in an aging nation with heavy consumption
of medical services, is the most striking feature of Japanese health care—
and one that other nations wish they could emulate. In fact, the secret
to Japan's low health care costs is simple: The system shafts doctors and
hospitals, paying some of the lowest fees on earth for medical treatment.
Of course, you really can't call this a secret; in fact, it's published in a
thick book—about the size of the Tokyo telephone directory—that
anybody can buy. This hefty volume, the *Shinryo Tensu Hyakumihyo*
("Quick Reference Guide to Medical Treatment Points"), sets forth
exactly what a doctor, therapist, or hospital will be paid for any treatment or medication. There are tens of thousands of different treatments
in the book: "throat swab," "application of plaster cast, ankle," "sutures,
outer arm," "X-ray, simple, neck region, rear," etc., etc. For almost all of
these, the price is extremely low, whether it's a simple office visit with
a family doctor (about $7), one night's stay in a four-bed hospital ward
($15, with meals and nursing care included), one night in a private room
at the hospital ($105, meals and care included), or a total shoulder ar-
throplasty. For virtually all forms of medical treatment, the prices in
Japan are far below average fees in other developed countries.

"In Japan, doctors don't get rich," Dr. Nakamichi, the famous orthopedist, told me that day in his clinic at Keio. "We make a decent
income. We have the pleasure of practicing our specialty, and helping

people who are in pain. But getting rich is not part of the expectation. With the prices we are paid, doctors are average earners." A Japanese general practitioner with a family practice in a big city might take home about $130,000 per year, significantly less than her counterpart in the United States. Specialists like Dr. Nakamichi generally earn less than $200,000 per year—again, far less than an American surgeon of similar renown could expect to earn. Like the doctors in France and Germany, Japanese physicians earn about as much as a midlevel corporate executive. They are comfortably middle class but generally not members of the country-club set.

The prices that Japanese insurers pay to doctors and hospitals are set every two years in a national negotiation between the Japanese Medical Association—the trade group representing doctors—and the national government's health ministry. The Fee Schedule that results from the biennial back-and-forth is the key governing tool of Japanese health care. "The doctors are private," says Professor Ikegami, the economist. "The insurance plans are mostly private. But the Ministry of Health and Welfare determines which treatments and drugs the insurance plans have to pay for, and negotiates the prices that insurance has to pay. So you have a multipayer system that works like a single-payer system. The single national Fee Schedule gives the ministry enormous power." In essence, Japan's market for medical services is a competitive free market operating under the firm hand of government regulation. This is something like the market for home telephone service in the United States. The phone companies are private firms, free to compete in the market, except on price. The price for basic land-line service is set by the local Public Service Commission or some other government regulator.

A good example of how this works in Japan is the price of a magnetic resonance imaging (MRI) scan. In the United States, a standard MRI scan of the head costs about $1,000 to $1,400. In Japan, the health ministry thinks that price is far too high. The fixed price for an

MRI of the head in Japan is ¥11,400, or $105. That's why Japan, with the highest per capita rate of MRI scans in the world, still spends less than most developed countries on health care; you can buy a lot of scans if the price is dirt-cheap. I once asked Professor Ikegami why doctors put up with this; why don't they just refuse to take MRI scans if the fee is so low? "The answer to that is the Fee Schedule," the economist replied. "There's only one payment scale in Japan. If a doctor won't accept the price in the schedule, he won't get any business. And he won't have the scans he needs to diagnose his patients. So the doctors accept the price."

In America, drug companies and medical device makers argue that they have to charge high prices to fund their research and development. But Japanese experience shows that tough cost controls tend to drive innovation, not stifle it. Because the permitted fee for an MRI scan is so low, for example, Japanese doctors went to the MRI manufacturers—Hitachi, Toshiba, etc.—and demanded a new line of compact, inexpensive MRI machines. The industry responded. Today, Japanese doctors and clinics can buy MRI scanners for around $150,000—about one-tenth the price of the bigger machines used in the United States. That helps keep prices down for the Japanese health care system. And the new line of cheap, simple MRI machines has been an export boon for the Japanese manufacturers, giving them a lock on the MRI market in poorer countries. These cut-price models perform the basic scanning job but don't have all the advanced features of top-of-the-line models generally used in the United States. So cost control not only keeps prices down; it also encourages innovation.

Still, there's a long-term price to be paid for keeping providers' prices low. Many Japanese hospitals today are severely underfunded. It is not just that they tend to be dumpy, gray concrete structures with sparse facilities and crowded spaces. Beyond that, the stiff cost-control regime limits the ability of doctors and private hospitals to incorporate expensive new techniques and equipment. The national association of private hospitals says that about 50 percent of hospitals and clinics in Japan are badly underfunded, with many on the verge of bankruptcy. Most of the innovation in Japanese medicine comes in the relatively small number of hospitals affiliated with major medical schools; thus it was not surprising that I found Dr. Nakamichi, the leading-edge orthopedic surgeon, at Keio Daigaku Hospital, part of the medical school at Keio University. The one saving grace for Japanese hospitals is that many of them were built, and are maintained, by big Japanese corporations to serve their employees. And these hospitals—which are open to everybody, regardless of the sponsoring company—can still depend on the company to cough up the money when it is time to build a new ward or install a new operating theater. But the corporate hospitals tend to be clustered in a few big cities; the hospitals in smaller towns and rural areas have to struggle along with a Fee Schedule that provides almost no margin for improvement.

In addition to setting prices, the biennial negotiation between the health ministry and the doctors' association also establishes which treatments and medication the insurance plans must pay for. This list tends to be expansive; Japanese health insurance covers a huge range of Chinese and Western medical services, including dental, psychiatric, and chiropractic care. The glaring exception, to Western eyes, is the plans' failure to cover pregnancy and childbirth. "Medical insurance should cover treatment for accident and disease," Dr. Ikegami explains, "but pregnancy is a natural condition of healthy women, so it is not insured." At first blush, this seems a foolish policy choice in a nation with a falling population that desperately needs to encourage young families to have children. In practice, almost all expectant mothers receive a "maternity grant" from the local government as soon as their pregnancy is diagnosed. The handout comes to $3,000 or so; that is roughly enough to pay for prenatal care, delivery, and postnatal care for mother and child.

THE BIG LOSERS in the Japanese health care system, the people who come out worst, are the providers of health care—doctors, nurses, therapists, and hospitals. That point came home to me one spring morning in Koshigaya, a sleepy, uncrowded Tokyo neighborhood, when I visited the Kono Medical Clinic, a nineteen-bed private hospital owned by Dr. Kono Hitoshi, a general practitioner, and his wife, Dr. Kono Keiko, an ophthalmologist. The six doctors at the clinic see about three hundred outpatients per day, and most nights there are twelve to fifteen inpatients staying in the hospital ward. Like much of Tokyo, the Kono clinic was erected after World War II, when Japan was rushing to rebuild its shattered cities and aesthetics didn't matter. It is a drab off-white concrete structure that looks like a small warehouse or an aging factory. The building sits on a small side street—an alley, really, so narrow that drivers have to fold in their outside mirrors to traverse it—about two blocks from the center of Koshigaya. In front of the building there's a ten-car parking lot for patients. And this lot is ruthless. Each of the parking spots has a thick metal bar that rests on the asphalt until a car pulls in. Then the bar snaps up and blocks the car; the driver can't get out of the lot until he pays a parking fee ($4 per hour).

Dr. Kono, a balding, round-faced man who wears a white doctor's jacket with his title on the pocket—*In-cho*, or "Head of Clinic"—is a jovial sort, with a ready smile and a steady supply of jokes. So I teased him about the parking fee at his clinic: Why would you charge for parking in a quiet neighborhood where anybody could park for free on the street a block away? "That's no laughing matter," Dr. Kono replied. "We sometimes make $100 in a day from that parking lot. And doctors in Japan don't make much money, so we have to figure out how to take in every yen we can get."

In fact, Dr. Kono told me, that struggle to break even is a daily fact

of life for a neighborhood doctor in Japan. His clinic is clean but spartan, with metal chairs, tile floors, white plaster walls, and a big room
full of aging file cabinets to hold his patients' records. A small, un-
adorned room with a brown vinyl bench is home to the clinic's MRI
scanner, one of the plain vanilla Toshiba models that cost about
$300,000. In the simple waiting room, where patients wait quietly on
long, backless benches until their names are called, there are a couple
of vending machines selling candy and yogurt drinks—another small
but steady source of income that is essential to the bottom line. The
waiting room tends to be full from early morning to midafternoon
each day, because almost all patients come to the clinic without an
appointment. "My patients feel they are entitled to see a doctor any
day they want to, so they just walk in," Dr. Kono told me with a wistful
sigh. "We have tried and tried to get them to call for appointments,
especially when they don't have any serious problem. But hardly
anybody calls ahead of time. And we can't keep them waiting very
long, either. There are other doctors and clinics in Koshigaya."

To prove how tough things can be for a Japanese medical practice,
Dr. Kono hauled out that fat volume—the Fee Schedule—that lists the
price he's paid for every treatment. "Look at this!" he said. "For a standard consultation, somebody has a bad cold or is worried about her
blood pressure, I get less than $20. Let's say an eight-year-old comes in
with an earache. I diagnose it, I give him an injection and a prescription,
and send him home. My fee is $10. If I admit somebody to the hospital,
in a four-bed room, the total fee we get, including dinner, is $15. For
an X-ray, I will be paid about $30. Who can live on that?" The notori-
ous Fee Schedule is fairly generous in reimbursing the doctor for making house calls—he can make as much as $400 for one visit if he brings
drugs and administers several tests in the patient's home. Accordingly,
Dr. Kono sets out once or twice a week in a special van, with a driver,
a pharmacist, and a medical technician, to make the rounds of elderly

patients in Koshigaya. It's clear that the home-bound patients welcome this attention, and Dr. Kono enjoys the visits as well.

Actually, Dr. Kono and his wife do fairly well at their clinic, earning a joint income of about $160,000 per year. That's roughly the average family income in Japan for a dual-income couple with college degrees. Unlike his American counterparts, Dr. Kono emerged from medical school with no student debt; the tuition was only $1,500 per year, and the local government helped pay it, as many municipal governments still do in Japan. When I asked him how much he pays annually for malpractice insurance, the doctor was stumped. "It's covered in my dues to the medical association," he said. "The dues are about $100 per month, but you also get the magazine and the directory for that." At the maximum, then, Dr. Kono and his nineteen-bed hospital are paying $1,200 per year for malpractice insurance, a smidgen of what a comparable clinic would pay in the United States. "I buy the insurance for peace of mind, but I don't think we need it," Dr. Kono said. In some forty years of operations, neither the Kono Medical Clinic nor any of its doctors has ever faced a malpractice suit.

Dr. Kono, like almost every doctor I've met in any country, likes to complain about the health care system and its failure to compensate him adequately. Still, he's not going to give up his clinic for some other line of work. Medicine is in his blood. The first Kono Medical Clinic was established by his grandfather in Tokyo's Tsugamo neighborhood before World War II. That clinic was destroyed in the firebombing of Tokyo in March of 1945. The family prudently fled Tokyo for a safer place to live; unfortunately, the safe haven they chose was the city of Hiroshima. When he was a child, Dr. Kono's mother told him about the day she saw the red glow from the atomic explosion.

The Kono family began rebuilding, with the rest of Japan, after the war. Dr. Kono's father built the new Kono Medical Clinic in, Koshigaya, then a farming section of Tokyo. The business prospered as

Koshigaya became an urban neighborhood. At its height, the clinic had thirty-nine beds and was nearly full most nights. Following the familiar footsteps, Kono Hitoshi went to medical school. He married Keiko, his med-school sweetheart, and the two of them came home to Koshigaya and the clinic. For all his gripes about a doctor's plight in contemporary Japan, he proudly notes that the couple's oldest daughter, Kono Makiko, is now in medical school.

Despite the Scrooge-like Fee Schedule and the intense competition among physicians, there has been no doctor shortage in Japan (although some rural areas have seen their doctors move to big cities recently). Families like the Konos, with four generations of physicians, are one reason. There's a strong cultural pattern of doctors' children following their parents to medical school; at some schools, the legacies make up about half the student body. Another factor is that physicians enjoy significant status in Japan's hierarchical society; this is true in most countries, but in Japan doctoring is a particularly prestigious line of work. As in Britain and the United States, there are countless movies and TV shows about brilliant, attractive doctors who diagnose and cure all manner of exotic ailments. Doctors and hospitals are also common subjects in the rich world of *manga,* the graphic novels—that is, comic books for grown-ups—that sell by the millions each week all over Japan. One of the all-time classics of the *manga* world was *Black Jack* (in Japanese, *Buraku-jaku*), a long-running medical soap opera created by the Ernest Hemingway of *manga,* author and illustrator Tezuka Osamu. The *Black Jack* books have been best sellers in Japan almost continuously since the 1960s. In its current manifestation, *New Black Jack,* the series concerns a young surgeon named Saito who teaches at a medical school— the comic book is full of detailed anatomical drawings of the colon, the scrotum, etc. In just about every episode, Dr. Saito saves lives with dramatic emergency operations. He also writes textbooks, gives public lectures about the evils of tobacco (the comics include detailed epidemiological charts of the Japanese population), and still finds time to romance a lovely and mysterious nurse who keeps trying to sneak a smoke when her doctor-boyfriend isn't looking. The result of all this glamour and romance is that bright young Japanese students, regardless of the dreaded Fee Schedule, still dream of becoming doctors. Or marrying them. "It's still true," Professor Ikegami explained, "that if a young woman calls home to tell her parents that she has become engaged to a wonderful man, the parents' pleasure is even greater if the daughter can add, 'And he's a doctor!'"

The high esteem for doctors is reflected in a traditional cultural practice in Japan that is officially frowned upon these days but still seems to exist: Patients tend to bring a present for their doctor, ranging from a box of golf balls to a magnum of sake to a tasteful white envelope with the physician's name brushed on the outside and a packet of cash inside. In the better stationery stores, you can buy special envelopes for this purpose, in soft, thick paper the color of heavy cream with "the honorable physician" written on them in elaborate calligraphy. This tradition dates back to premodern times, when a physician in China or Japan had a Confucian obligation to use his skills to treat people and was not expected to demand a fee. To express their gratitude, patients provided a more or less voluntary gratuity. Some historians argue that this Confucian mind-set is one reason doctors' fees are so low today.

That artifact of an older society was one of many cultural idiosyncrasies that our family dealt with when we lived in Japan. Thanks to the negotiated Fee Schedule, of course, the prices at the doctor's office always seemed low—so low that I often wondered whether it would be appropriate to hand over some extra cash as a gift to the physician. To give or not to give? In my doctor's office in Tokyo, there was a sign on the wall clearly stating that the doctor's fee for each treatment, and the share of the fee that I had to co-pay, were set by law: HONORABLE PATIENTS ARE RESPECTFULLY REQUESTED TO PAY NO MORE THAN THE FEE, it said. But I did sometimes see a patient, particularly an older person, carrying one of those cream-colored envelopes into the doctor's office. To make things even more perplexing, the first Japanese doctor I ever went to, years ago, refused to accept any payment at all. After he treated me the first time, Dr. Suzuki said that he remembered various acts of kindness by American GIs during the postwar occupation of Japan; he wanted to demonstrate his gratitude to America, he said firmly, by treating this particular American for free. In a reversal of Confucian tradition, Dr. Suzuki even sent a gift to our house after we left his office—a handsome vase, which stands on our mantel to this day.

There was another clash of cultures one day when I went to our neighborhood doctor with flu and a bad fever. I was ushered into an office; a nurse bowed to me and handed me a glass thermometer. I put it under my tongue, sat in a chair, and pulled out a magazine. It was clear from the look of horror on the nurse's face that something was terribly wrong. But what? Given the gap in stature between a deferential apprentice nurse and a senior foreign journalist, it was just about impossible for this young Japanese woman to tell the older American man that he had done something absurd. So we just sat there, the two of us, through a long, uncomfortable, but polite silence—until the doctor himself came in, laughed at our predicament, and told me that a Japanese thermometer was meant to be inserted under the armpit.

Nonetheless, our American family did fine with the Japanese medical system. We never had to wait for an appointment, the doctors were gentle and knowledgeable, and the earnest, polite office staff always acted as if treating our son's case of flu or mumps or poison ivy was the most important medical concern in the entire Japanese archipelago. At the Kitasato Clinic, an impressive new hospital near our home, there was a poster in the reception area that set forth "Our Hospital's Mission." I liked it so much, I copied the whole text into my notebook one day:

1. We will welcome you with a smiling face, warm sympathy, and soft language.

2. As Dr. Kitasato, our founder, often said: We know our patients are worried. We want to give them a sense of assurance about their health.

3. We will do all in our power to protect your privacy and dignity.

4. Preserving your life and health is the reason this hospital exists.

As in other Japanese business establishments, everyone at my doctor's office was relentlessly courteous. They bowed to me; they thanked me for honoring their humble clinic with my esteemed patronage; they always referred to me as "Reido-sama," "the highly honorable Mr. Reid"; they apologized profusely for keeping us waiting, even on those occasions when we were ushered right in to the doctor with no waiting at all. I got similar effusions each year around my birthday, when a letter would arrive from the government of Shibuya, our section of Tokyo. "Dear Highly Honorable Mr. Reid," the annual missive began. "Please accept our humble apologies for intruding on your busy daily life, but we would respectfully urge you to have your esteemed body checked in an annual physical exam. Your comprehensive physical examination will be free, at any doctor's clinic in Shibuya, if your heavy schedule will permit you to complete it within thirty days of your birthday." This was too good a deal to pass up, and I always took advantage of it. I remembered that free annual physical some years later when we lived in Britain and the National Health Service refused to give me a free physical exam. The Japanese had decided that an exam was worth the price in terms of prevention; the British system had concluded precisely the opposite.

One medical problem the Japanese doctors always detected in those free annual physicals was my bum right shoulder. I was urged to do something about it and was eventually steered to Dr. Nakamichi, the prominent surgeon who saw me in his office the same day I called him.

I first had to navigate the complex maze of the teeming reception lobby at the Keio Daigaku Hospital, one of Tokyo's major medical centers. Eventually, I made my way through the drab gray hallways to the Orthopedic Surgery Department. (In Japanese, "orthopedics" is called *seikei,* written with two characters that mean "aligning the frame.") In a drab gray waiting room I sat on a backless bench of cracked vinyl until a nurse called, "The highly honorable Thomas Reid." I entered the doctor's office—basically, just a cubicle with two old chairs and a small gray desk. The doctor seemed harried; he had already seen twenty patients that day, he said, and there were a dozen or more waiting after me. While we were discussing my shoulder problem, the surgeon looked up the condition on his computer—something no other doctor, in any country, had done—and discussed the possible treatments listed there. He first described something he called "Chee She Emmu," which mystified me until I realized this was the Japanese pronunciation of the English abbreviation TCM, for "traditional Chinese medicine"; this approach includes herbal massage and acupuncture. Japanese insurance would pay for that. A physical therapist with an exercise regime could help, he said. Japanese insurance would pay for that. He could also try a monthly steroid injection, which would alleviate pain and might lead to greater movement. Japanese insurance would pay for that. And of course, he could perform the total shoulder arthroplasty that my American orthopedist had suggested. Dr. Nakamichi thought the surgery was not the best solution for me; shoulder-replacement surgery is indicated mainly to alleviate pain, he said, while my problem was mainly stiffness. But if I chose the operation, Japanese insurance would pay for that, too. "Think about it, and call me," the doctor said, and then the nurse was nudging me, politely but firmly, out of the office. "We have a waiting room full of people yet to see today," she explained.

In that crowded, dingy, but ever-so-polite clinic, I saw both sides of Japanese medicine. There was instant access to fine doctors, a considerable range of choice for the patients, and a private insurance system that seemed to cover just about everything. There was also a sense of a medical infrastructure that was overstretched and pinching pennies. In a sense, that makes Japanese medicine the mirror image of America. Our country spends too much on health care and gets too little in return; Japan gets lots of health care but probably spends too little to make its excellent system sustainable.

SEVEN

The UK: Universal Coverage, No Bills

LORD WILLIAM BEVERIDGE AND NYE BEVAN CAME FROM opposite ends of the British Empire and opposite poles of the British class divide. Beveridge, the aristocratic social reformer, grew up in a Darjeeling mansion with seventeen rooms and twenty-six servants (not counting his nanny). Bevan, the pugnacious miner and union agitator turned politician, shared a four-room cottage in South Wales with nine siblings who would have loved to be employed as servants but were instead destined to a life of hard labor in the coal pits. What brought these two men together, midway through the twentieth century, was the conviction that a modern state must provide medical care to everybody, sick or well, young or old, rich or poor.

The British National Health Service, the system that Beveridge designed and Bevan muscled into existence sixty years ago, is dedicated to the proposition that nobody should ever have to pay a medical bill. In the NHS, there is no insurance premium to pay, no co-payment, no fee at all, whether you drop by the GP's office with a cold or receive a quadruple bypass from the nation's top cardiac surgeon. The doctor's bill is paid by the government, and the patient never even thinks about it. There are private health insurance plans in the United Kingdom, but few people bother with them. Nine out of ten Britons get all their health care from the NHS. People go their entire lives without ever paying a doctor or hospital bill; in Britain, this is considered normal.

The Brits do pay for medical care, of course. They pay through a network of taxes that would make Americans cringe; the sales tax in the UK is 17.5 percent on anything you buy, while income and social security taxes are higher than America's in every income bracket. The Brits pay by forgoing treatments and medications that the NHS won't provide. They pay by waiting in lines for care in a system that is sometimes overstretched. But the single national system, with minimal paperwork and no billing, has proven to be an unusually cost-efficient means of providing quality health care to everybody. It cares for roughly one-fifth the population of the United States but spends only one-fifteenth of the U.S. health care bill. And yet the results are good: Britain has lower child mortality, longer healthy life spans, and better recovery rates from most major diseases than does the United States.

Beyond all that, the Beveridge-Bevan system has been a clear political success. The people who provide care in the NHS are enormously proud of their system and the work they do. The people who receive care from the NHS are among the most satisfied medical customers on earth. When our family lived in Britain, we, too, were satisfied with the care we got from the NHS—most of the time. We sometimes had to wait long weeks to see a specialist, which was galling. On the other hand, we never had to wait long weeks for the insurance company to pay the doctor bill, because (have I mentioned this?) there was no bill. When it came to my bad shoulder, however—as we'll see shortly—the National Health Service did zilch. I was instructed, in classic stiff-upper-lip style, to adjust to the stiffness in my shoulder and get on with life.

Free nationalized health care is such a basic part of British life today that not even the iron lady of British conservatism, Margaret Thatcher, ever dared take on the NHS. Her Conservative Party privatized the coal mines, the railroads, the telephones, the water supply—but not health care. "Margaret would never touch the NHS," said Nigel Lawson, who was her chancellor of the exchequer (basically, budget director). "In Britain today, the NHS is the closest thing we have to a religion." When Conservative David Cameron was elected prime minister in 2010, he promised severe cutbacks in government spending—except for the NHS, where he pledged to spend more.

The Beveridge Model of health care has been adopted, with variations, by nations around the world, democracies and dictatorships alike. A system in which government owns the hospitals, pays the doctors, buys the medicine, and covers all the bills would probably come pretty close to what American politicians have in mind when they deplore "socialized medicine." But America, too, has copied the NHS model—to provide treatment for tens of millions of Native Americans, military personnel, dependents, and veterans. With government doctors in government clinics dispensing government drugs (and no bills for the patients to pay), the U.S. Department of Veterans Affairs is one of the purest examples anywhere of the Beveridge Model at work. If this is un-American, why did we choose it for America's military veterans?

IT'S NOT SURPRISING THAT Nye Bevan would spend much of his adult life fighting to provide decent medical care to his countrymen. As a boy in the Welsh coalfields at the dawn of the twentieth century, Bevan saw what could happen to decent families when sickness struck and there was no access to medicine. Although his own family had a steady income and owned its little home, the young Bevan saw four of his siblings die of illness while still children, and watched his father succumb painfully to a long ailment, pneumoconiosis, that was not treated.

But William Beveridge's burning commitment to equal care for all had no such childhood roots. The son of a senior official of the British Raj, Beveridge had a pampered upbringing, first in Darjeeling and later—when his mother refused to face another scorching Indian summer—in a country mansion on twelve acres near the white cliffs of Dover. The boy had all the care, medical and otherwise, that wealth and privilege could provide. He was sent to one of those Victorian boarding schools that believed in building character through cold showers and Latin prose composition, but he escaped those hardships when he enrolled at Oxford in 1897. There he acquired the nickname "Drink"—evidently a play on his last name, not a reference to his leisure habits—and spent his university years considering the various professions open to a young man of his stature.[1]

One standard vocation for Oxford men at the time was the clergy. Young Beveridge spurned that route, explaining to his sister that "I believe neither in Heaven, which would be insipid, nor in Hell, which would be ridiculous." A tutor suggested that William follow in his father's footsteps with a career in the civil service; the young man concluded that this work would be "neither interesting nor remunerative." On graduating, he entered the chambers of a London barrister to study law; he left a few months later, telling his disappointed mother that an attorney's life appeared "solitary, self-centered, and intellectually trivial."

And then Beveridge found the work that would become his career: social reform. Urged by an Oxford don to look into "the mystery of poverty," he took a job in 1903 at a settlement house—basically, an inner-city charity—in the slums of East London. There, the fortunate son of the Raj was stunned to learn how rotten life could be for the ragged, hungry, and sickly families of the other half. He saw conditions so ghastly that he would never forget them. He met children eager to learn but too hungry or too sick to attend school; he met men willing to work but incapacitated by illness; he saw women dying in agony in childbirth—and all of them utterly cut off from medical care. Beveridge began writing newspaper columns urging revolutionary ideas: free school lunches for starving children, public-works jobs for their parents, unemployment compensation. The young social worker's most daring proposal was downright radical: "a national health service for prevention and comprehensive treatment, available to all."[2]

For the next four decades, Beveridge pursued those goals as an officer of countless charities and official boards: the Stepney Distress Committee, the School Dinner Association, the Children's Country Holiday Fund, the Family Endowment Society, the Poor Law Commission, the Social Insurance Society, and many more. By the 1940s, he was a famous figure, the paradigm of a familiar British type, the "reforming intellectual." He was a driven man, right to the end; his last words, enunciated clearly from his death bed at the age of eighty-four, showed that the aging social reformer was still haunted by the memory of those sick men on the East London streets. "I have a thousand things to do," he said, and died. But by then—Beveridge died in 1963—he had seen his most dramatic innovation develop into a cherished element of British life.

Beveridge's opportunity to reform health care on a national scale came in the early 1940s. After the United States and the UK had turned the tide in World War II and seemed on course to defeat the Nazis, Britain's leaders began thinking ahead to the domestic programs that would be required to rebuild the country after the war. When Winston Churchill's coalition government created an official Committee on Social Insurance and Allied Services, the obvious choice to lead the effort was the prominent aristocratic reformer William Beveridge. The committee was staffed with senior experts from the ministries of health, labor, pensions, and so forth, but in fact, its work was largely a one-man operation. Beveridge wrote every word of the committee's report. Naturally, it endorsed nearly all the social reforms he had championed over the decades. But the centerpiece was the concept of a government-run National Health Service, open to everyone. As Beveridge planned it, health care would be free to all at the doctor's office or hospital; payment would come not from medical fees or insurance companies but through general taxation.

When it came out in 1942, with the people of Britain just gaining the confidence to think about a bright new world after the war, the Beveridge plan was an explosive success. At a time when a popular new book might sell twenty thousand copies in a year, the Beveridge Report—officially, *Social Insurance and Allied Services*—sold one hundred thousand in a month. The military distributed copies to every British fighting man to enhance morale. The press was euphoric. The report and its author became so immensely popular that the Rockefeller Foundation brought Beveridge to America, where he gave one hundred speeches on his plan and saw the report sell a further fifty thousand copies. Back home, he was honored with a lordship—he became, officially, Baron Beveridge of Tuggal. He served for years in the House of Lords, but Baron Beveridge was never really a politician. He lacked the cunning, and the clout, to make his bold policy proposal a legal reality.

THAT JOB FELL INSTEAD to the obstreperous but cunning Welsh coal miner Aneurin "Nye" Bevan. The grandson, son, nephew, and brother of coal miners, Bevan was born in a cottage a short walk from the pit at Tredegar, a mining valley flanked on all sides by other coaling valleys. His parents gave their children traditional Welsh names and a standard Welsh upbringing: a few years of school before they were sent to work in the pits. Young Aneurin (pronounced Ah-NY-rin) became a full-time coal miner on his thirteenth birthday, in 1910. "There is a tiredness that leads to stupor," he wrote years later, recalling his early days in the Tredegar pit. "There is the tiredness of the miner, particularly the boy of 14 who falls asleep over his meals and wakes up hours later to find the evening has gone and there is nothing before him but bed and another day's wrestling with inert matter."[3]

What distinguished young Nye Bevan from the other adolescent miners was a seething anger over his plight, and a determination to fight it. The young militant joined the South Wales Miners' Federation and quickly moved into the union's leadership ranks. At the union library in Tredegar, he studied Karl Marx and the American socialist Eugene V. Debs and concluded that "equality under socialism" was the answer to the basic unfairness of the British class system. A ferocious advocate, despite a lingering stutter, he became a prominent voice for the miners' cause. At the age of thirty-two, he was elected to the House of Commons as the Labour Party candidate from the neighboring valley of Ebbw Vale.

The belligerent member from Ebbw Vale proved just as much a fighter in Parliament as in the pits. For most of Bevan's political career, his role was to attack the ruling Conservative Party, and he took to it with vituperative relish. Bevan's favorite Tory target was Winston Churchill, even during the years when Churchill was lionized as the leader of the anti-Nazi cause. While global radio audiences tuned in to hear Churchill's inspiring speeches, Bevan brushed off the prime minister's rhetoric as "turgid, wordy, dull, prosaic, and almost invariably empty." (Churchill, for his part, dismissed Bevan as a "squalid nuisance.")[4]

And then Bevan got the chance to move off the back benches. In the summer of 1945, just weeks after the surrender of Germany, the British people showed their gratitude to their wartime leader by voting his Conservatives out of office. The new Labour prime minister, Clement Attlee, offered Nye Bevan a place in his cabinet as minister of health. The determined socialist immediately declared that his chief priority in the new job would be to give Britons socialized medicine—that is, the free, universal, nationalized health care system set forth in the famous Beveridge Report. Bevan pledged to "take the money out of medicine" by enacting the Beveridge Model.

It was to be Aneurin Bevan's greatest battle, but he started with considerable advantages. The Beveridge Report had caught the public fancy; any pro-Beveridge politician was riding a wave of popular support. During the years of total war, much of British medicine had been managed by a central Emergency Hospital Service, so the idea of a single national system was not unheard of. Still, the minister of health got into a furious fight with the British Medical Association, representing the nation's general practitioners. They had always been private practitioners and had no inclination whatsoever to become salaried civil servants. Meanwhile, the existing health insurance programs, known as "friendly societies," were not at all friendly toward a nationalized system likely to put them out of business. Bevan, true to his nature, took on both foes with free-swinging gusto.

But he also proved adroit at compromise, and his negotiations produced a modus operandi still found in the National Health Service today. Bevan decided that all hospitals—municipal, charity, and private—would be nationalized as part of the NHS. The specialists working in the hospitals—surgeons, orthopedists, radiologists, and so on—would all be government employees. To win the backing of these specialists, Bevan agreed that they could continue to see patients on their own time, and charge fees. This essentially created a private medical system alongside the NHS; but Bevan predicted, correctly, that the private system would never amount to more than a smidgen of the free public service. (Today, private care constitutes about 3 percent of British medicine.) Next, in a crucial concession to the British Medical Association, he agreed that general practitioners could remain private operators, treating patients in their own offices but receiving their fee directly from the NHS. Next, Bevan told the insurance industry that it could still market medical policies to any customers who chose not to use the NHS. These detours from pure socialized medicine did not sit well with an organization of left-wing doctors known as the Socialist Medical Association, but Bevan resisted their pressure. He had secured his main goals—universal coverage, with no medical bills—and that was enough. On July 5, 1948, the National Health Service opened its doors, free to all comers.

From its earliest days, the NHS faced a problem that still persists six decades later: When you make medical care free, people tend to use a lot of medical care. The NHS exceeded its budget in its first year of operation and in most years thereafter.[5] Bevan fought tooth and nail for his service and usually won, because the NHS was the Labour government's most popular initiative. Eventually, though, officials at the treasury demanded some contribution from patients to offset the costs of health care. Bevan, the health minister, agreed to a nominal charge on prescriptions, as long as it did not apply to children or the elderly. But he drew the line at any other fees. In 1951, when the Labour government decided to charge patients for spectacles and false teeth, Bevan resigned his ministry, arguing (incorrectly, as it turned out) that this would inevitably lead to cash charges for office visits and hospital treatment in the NHS. He returned to the back benches of Parliament and spent his remaining years fulminating, as usual, against Conservative governments. Today, most of his contentious rhetoric is long forgotten; Aneurin Bevan is remembered for one thing. In July of 2008, when the UK celebrated a proud, boisterous sixtieth birthday party for the health service, marchers paraded past Big Ben carrying banners with Nye Bevan's picture and the caption FATHER OF THE NHS.

ENTERING ITS SEVENTH DECADE, the British National Health Service is a mammoth operation. With more than a million full-time staffers, it is the biggest employer in Europe. It owns two thousand hospitals, about ten times as many as Hospital Corporation of America, the world's biggest private hospital company. The British press gives the health service the kind of blanket coverage that the U.S. media reserve for Britney Spears. Most newspapers and news shows have at least one NHS story every day. There are TV shows about the NHS, both fictional and documentary, virtually every night of the week; the American hit *ER* was derived from the hugely popular British TV drama *Casualty*. Mills & Boon, the nation's biggest publisher of romance novels, has a division that specializes in NHS love stories (such as *Virgin Midwife, Playboy Doctor* and *Emergency: Wife Needed*); the books sell like mad.

But the structure of this vast organization is still pretty much what the architect, Beveridge, and the builder, Bevan, had in mind. The NHS still provides medical care for everybody in the country, with no fee at the point of service. In theory, there is a charge for prescriptions (about $10); but since this fee is waived for children, anyone over sixty, pregnant women, and the chronically ill, about 85 percent of all the drugs in Britain are dispensed for free. Most people still have to pay for eyeglasses, contact lenses, false teeth, and some dental bills. Contrary to Nye Bevan's warning, though, the principle of paying for medical treatment has never expanded into a general system of fees. In the late 1990s, the British Medical Association proposed a standard co-pay of £10 ($15) per office visit, to be shared by the doctors and the NHS. The press and the public reacted with such outrage that the proposal was relegated instantly to the rubbish bin.

To keep its service free, the NHS strives mightily to keep its costs low—and in fact, it is recognized by experts around the world as one of the most cost-efficient health care plans ever devised. It is a model for any country that wants to provide quality care at low cost. One key reason, of course, is that no-fee funding mechanism. With no bills, no billing offices, no bureaucracy needed to file or review insurance claims, the administrative costs at the NHS are small—about one-fifth those in the United States. Beyond that, the British system uses various other mechanisms to keep a lid on expenses.

For the NHS, the first line of defense in cost control is the nationwide network of general practitioners, who have a powerful gatekeeping role. Everybody who wants access to NHS treatment—which is to say, everybody in Britain—has to register with a general practitioner. People have a broad choice in picking a primary doctor, but most just go to the closest "surgery"—that's British for a doctor's office—in their neighborhood. If you want to see a "consultant"—that's British for a medical specialist—you first have to go to your GP for a recommendation. Since many complaints can be managed just fine by a GP in the local clinic, this is a smart way to save the time and cost of expensive visits to specialists in the hospital. Indeed, the gatekeeper system is so effective at controlling costs that many U.S. health insurance plans have imposed the same requirement.

True to Bevan's original compromise, the GPs are independent businesspeople, not government employees. But most of them have only one source of payment: the NHS. A general practitioner is paid by a system known as capitation—that is, she gets a set fee for each person registered with her practice. This creates a clear economic incentive for the doctor to practice preventive medicine—another proven money-saver for any health care system.

"You know, the NHS pay me for the people on my list whether they come into the surgery or not," explained Dr. Ahmed Badat, an imposing six-footer with sleek black hair and a fifty-two-inch waist who was my GP. "So why do I want them in here? My message is: 'Look, mate: Don't get sick.' Some people I don't see for three years, five years. When they come in, no matter what it's for, I take their bloods and their urine and listen to their chest and put them on the scales. I want to know if they've got any problem, maybe they haven't noticed. Because it is my interest, see, to keep them healthy." As in most

British GP clinics, Dr. Badat's waiting room is wallpapered with NHS posters pushing preventive care: "MENINGITIS CAN KILL! RING 020 8753 1081 TO LEARN THE SYMPTOMS." "SIGN UP HERE FOR LIVING WELL WITH DIABETES—A FREE ONE-DAY WORKSHOP." "ASK AT RECEPTION ABOUT FREE NICOTINE REPLACEMENT THERAPY." "KNOWING ABOUT CERVICAL CANCER COULD SAVE YOUR DAUGHTER'S LIFE." During the flu shot months of fall and winter, the nurses at the Badat surgery all wear bright red pins that say, ASK ME ABOUT A FREE FLU JAB.

The most notorious cost-control tool in Britain's system is the dreaded "queue"—that is, the waiting list. Even when the gatekeeper agrees that you need to see a consultant, it can take weeks or months to get an appointment. In the late 1990s, when our family first moved to Britain, the newspapers had horrendous tales of NHS nontreatment, of patients left on a gurney in a hospital hallway for days because no bed was available. One notorious case involved a mother whose general practitioner spotted symptoms of throat cancer. He referred her to a hospital for consultation. She was put in the queue to see the specialist but had to wait so long for an appointment that, by the time her cancer was confirmed, it had grown too big to be removed. The resulting tabloid headline—MUM DIED IN THE QUEUE—was not precisely accurate, but it captured the core truth of the case.

American politicians regularly bring up this aspect of British health care as evidence that "socialized medicine" doesn't work. But that line of criticism, once valid, is somewhat out of date today. Under intense political pressure, Prime Minister Tony Blair and his successor, Gordon Brown, poured large sums into the NHS in this century specifically to reduce the waiting lists. NHS statistics suggest that this has made a major difference; waiting lists are much shorter than they were, say, fifteen years ago. But some people still have to wait, particularly for procedures that the NHS considers elective. In the fall of 2007, Dr. Badat told me how long his patients typically stay in the queue for specific complaints: "If you need a hernia repair, and there's no acute pain, I think it's about three months. Varicose veins is about six months. But if it's acute, that's different. We are much faster now. Any suspected cancer, seen by the consultant within two weeks. Any cardiac, we get you in the hospital the same day. If you got chest pain, I send you to cardiac within an hour."

The American physicians Thomas S. Bodenheimer and Kevin Grumbach studied the medical literature about NHS queues and summarized it this way:

> Primary and preventive care are not rationed, and average waiting times to see a GP are probably no longer than for similar appointments in many parts of the United States. Even some high-tech services (e.g., radiation therapy for cancer and bone marrow transplantation) are performed at the same rates as in the United States. But waiting times to see consultants for non-urgent problems may be substantial, and 38% of patients wait more than four months for elective surgeries.[6]

Finally, the NHS controls its budget by controlling the range of medications, tests, and procedures it will pay for. This kind of "rationing" takes place in every health care system; in the United States, such decisions are generally made in private, by insurance companies. But in Britain, with a public health care system that is a constant focus of public attention, the decisions about what treatment will be available— decisions that are literally life-and-death choices for many patients—are public. Should a ninety-four-year-old patient get a hip replacement? Should every man over fifty get a blood test for prostate cancer? Should a terminal cancer patient get the newest experimental treatment, because it just might work? Should a healthy reporter who wants to play golf again be given a total shoulder arthroplasty? The government office that answers those questions in Britain is called the National Institute for Health and Clinical Excellence. Everybody knows the outfit, though, by its acronym, NICE.

Naturally, headline writers in the newspapers find it almost impossible to resist puns on this name, particularly when NICE has decided that some expensive drug designed to fight cancer or AIDS will not be provided. A typical case involved Ann Marie Rogers, a pub waitress and mother of three in Swindon who contracted the HER-2 form of breast cancer. The NHS gave her surgery, chemotherapy, and radiotherapy. But she had read on the Internet that a drug called Herceptin could treat breast cancer without the discomfort of chemicals or radiation. When she asked for a prescription, the system turned her down. A study at NICE had concluded that Herceptin was not an effective treatment for her particular form of cancer; another factor may have been the price, about $36,000 per year for one patient. Rogers and her family went to court (in vain) to fight this ruling, and the tabloids jumped at the story: "Not So NICE—Mum Left to Fight Cancer Without a Pill."

When I asked the folks at NICE about that case, they didn't flinch. "That's exactly what NICE are here for," said Lucy Betterton, an associate director at the agency's headquarters. "There is a set amount of money in the NHS system, and somebody has to decide what it should and should not be spent on." The reason NICE gets pummeled in the press, she said, is that it is a government agency that operates transparently. "When we make an unpopular decision, it is out there for all to see. If you say to people, should there be an agency like NICE to make sure our health funds are spent wisely, they say yes. But if it's a kind mum who is turned down, the press splash it, you know: 'NICE is not nice!'"

The NHS can generally skate past this kind of criticism, because of the strong popular support for the system. Since everybody in Britain has a stake in the health service, there's a common political will to accept the harsh decisions it sometimes has to make. Because the NHS budget covers everybody, the money saved on one patient can be used to treat another. Declining to operate on a sick grandmother means there is more money available to treat sick children. Accordingly, protests about denied coverage tend to be muted. In the U.S. system, that trade-off doesn't apply; if an American insurance company refuses to pay $36,000 for Herceptin for one of its clients, the money saved is likely used to enhance profits.

WHEN OUR FAMILY LIVED in Britain, in the first years of the twenty-first century, we encountered all those cost-saving mechanisms within the NHS. Still, our overall impression was positive. For the standard kind of medical problems that a normal family encounters—flu, colds, rashes, intestinal complaints, eye exams, and the occasional broken bone or sprain—the NHS doctors performed on par with any treatment we have had in the United States. And all for free.

In a sense, our relationship with the NHS was love at first sight. In those first days after we moved to London, we found a lot to love. The lush green parks, the cheery pubs, the bustling street markets, the majestic cathedrals, the sweet voices of the boy choirs (and, more recently, girl choirs) inside those cathedrals, the roomy black cabs, the red double-decker buses—it all won our hearts. We found it much harder, though, to love the prices of things in the United Kingdom, with everything running about one and a half to three times as much as it costs in the United States. Adding injury to the insult was the stunning sales tax—a 17.5 percent tax tacked on to every purchase, far higher than the combined city and state sales tax in any American state. I kept wondering: Why do the Brits put up with a tax that high?

And then, barely a week after we arrived in the UK, our youngest daughter woke up with a painfully infected ear, bright red and swollen like a chestnut. We could guess the cause—it must have been that dubious ear-piercing shop in one of the charming street markets—but had no idea how to fix the problem. We had barely unpacked our suitcases and certainly hadn't had time to find a local doctor. Feeling desperate, we piled into a roomy black cab and asked to go the nearest hospital. Within minutes, we were in the emergency (that is, "casualty") ward at St. Mary's Hospital, an ancient, much-the-worse-for-wear institution on Praed Street, just down from Paddington Station. St. Mary's on Praed Street was the place where Sir Alexander Fleming discovered penicillin in 1928; it looked as if nobody had painted the walls since then. After a quarter-hour's wait there, a gentle nurse and an authoritative doctor took command of our daughter's case. They carefully removed the offending earring, reduced the swelling, treated the infection (with a form of penicillin), and offered polite but firm instruction on the right way to care for pierced ears.

Our daughter—and her parents—felt an enormous sense of relief. I pulled out my checkbook (that is, "chequebook") and waited for the bill. I knew this treatment was going to be costly—emergency rooms always are—but frankly, I was perfectly willing to pay for the excellent and reassuring medical care we had received. The nurse, evidently accustomed to American patients, smiled at my mistake. "You can put away your cheques," she said, crisply and proudly. "There won't be a bill to pay. We do it a bit differently here. In the National Health Service, we don't charge for medical treatment." With that, she sent us home.

Had the same minor medical crisis occurred at home, we would have received the same level of professional treatment. But we would have received something else along with it: a pile of bills. Having had a similar experience with emergency wards in the United States, I would expect that treatment like we got at St. Mary's in London would have brought bills of about $200 from the hospital, $150 or so from the doctor, and $100 from some lab technician. And I would likely have faced a three-month battle with an insurance company trying to get the bills paid. In Britain, there was no need to argue with the insurance company over the bill, because there was no bill (and, consequently, no insurance company). As we left the hospital, my wife said quietly, "Now I see why we pay that 17.5 percent."

In the aging but efficient casualty ward at St. Mary's Hospital, our family had come face to face with the Beveridge Model of health care, as implemented by Nye Bevan. We saw the pride and the powerful sense of service in the NHS staff, and we saw the run-down physical plant of a health system that is always stretched for funds. Mainly, we saw good medical treatment, for free. After that experience, we were committed to the NHS, even though my company provided decent health insurance that would have paid for private care.

The availability and quality of the care we had in Britain were about equal to what we had at home—better, in one sense, in that British doctors still make house calls. We generally got to see the doctor on the day we called. The doctor's surgery down the street from our house had a notice on the wall, warning, THE AVERAGE CONSULTATION SHOULD LAST 10 MINUTES. This seemed rather brief, although the British doctors never gave me the feeling that I was being rushed out the door. When I got back to the United States, I began timing my sessions with my American GP; generally, face-to-face time with Dr. Holder ran about ten minutes.

Thanks to the dictates of those cost-conscious researchers at NICE, our family found the NHS less inclined than American doctors to do tests and X-rays. The Brits wouldn't even give me an annual physical; Dr. Badat, the stout family doctor, told me that NHS economists had decided that the potential savings did not justify the cost, at least for basically healthy patients. Because the NHS puts so much emphasis on preventive care—and pays the doctors extra to provide it—many of the tests in a physical exam are routinely carried out when you go to the doctor. So the system doesn't pay for a separate physical on top of the routine testing. "You want a physical?" Dr. Badat laughed at me. "Here's a number. Ring them up. You pay them 350 quid [$500], you get a physical, private service." In the United States, a man my age is routinely given a PSA test to check for prostate cancer. I was never able to convince the NHS to do this for me. Even when I was sent to a neighborhood hospital for a blood test, the doctor declined to check the spot on the form calling for a PSA test as well. I argued about this with Dr. Badat. "The NHS don't think PSA is a proper indicator of cancer," he said. "It is not really accurate for disease of the prostate. So it is not considered cost-effective." To me, of course, this test would be considered extremely effective if it spotted a cancer in my body early enough to be treated. The determining factor, though, is not the individual's need to cover every base but NICE's concern to provide cost-effective medical care to an entire population.

On the other hand, the NHS gatekeeper did agree that I should get a colonoscopy to check for colon cancer, because of a family history of this disease. And once that decision was made, the system pulled out all the stops—letters, educational pamphlets, phone calls—to be sure I understood the test and the dietary preparations necessary before I went to the hospital for it. To my relief, the test showed nothing. But for the rest of my residence in Britain, the hospital wrote me every year to schedule a repeat colonoscopy. "If you have a risk of that cancer, of course the NHS are going to test for it," Dr. Badat explained to me. "It's better for you, and for the NHS, if they find it and treat it early." In the United States, depending on the hospital and the insurance plan, this procedure costs a patient between $100 and $2,400. In the UK, of course, my repeated colonoscopies cost me nothing.

But the National Health Service provided no service at all for my sore right shoulder.

I explained the history and symptoms of my shoulder problem to Dr. Badat. I showed him how restricted the movement was, told him about the occasional pain. He looked carefully at the X-rays and did the same kind of palpation that doctors had been doing for years. He tested the range of motion in my joint and the muscular strength. He looked over the NICE guidelines for treatment of shoulder ailments. And then he explained what would happen if I tried to get that shoulder surgically repaired in Britain's National Health Service. He was blunt.

"My job, you know, is to assess your medical problem," he began, "decide whether you need a consultant, which kind of specialist, all that. And I could get you an appointment with an orthopod, a shoulder man. In your state—no acute problem—the wait will be two months, three months. And the consultant will look you over and say, 'We don't do shoulder arthroplasty in the NHS unless there's a serious disability. You are living your normal life without much impairment. So it's not indicated.'" Dr. Badat sort of chuckled at the thought of it. "And then you can come back here to my surgery. And then I can send you to another consultant if you want. Another two, three months. And that bloke will say the same thing. And then you come back here again, and I'll tell you that you can get some physio [physical therapy] if you develop acute pain. Or you can get the operation privately and pay for it yourself. And that's what's going to happen in the NHS."

In other words, nothing was going to happen in the NHS. The operation that my American surgeon suggested without a moment's hesitation was a nonstarter in the British system. This result was not totally crazy; other doctors, in the United States and around the world, had told me I might not be a good candidate for a procedure as drastic as a total shoulder arthroplasty. But in Britain, I had the feeling that it was the system, not my medical condition, that made the surgery "not indicated." For that matter, a lot of things that are standard operating procedure in the United States—at least, for patients with adequate health insurance—are simply "not indicated" in the UK. "Overall, a striking characteristic of British medicine is its economy," wrote Drs. Bodenheimer and Grumbach, the American researchers. "British physicians simply do less of everything—perform fewer surgeries, prescribe fewer medications, and order fewer X-rays."[7]

Like most people in Britain, our family's chief interaction with the NHS came in visits to the GP. But then, most doctors in Britain—about 60 percent—are general practitioners. In the specialist-heavy United States, about 35 percent of doctors are general practitioners, and organizations like the American College of Physicians routinely deplore the shortage of medical students who choose to go into primary care. It's not hard to understand, though, why Britain has so many more doctors who choose a general practice. In contrast to most industrialized countries, the GPs in Britain generally make more money than the specialists—on average, about twice as much. In a generally socialized medical system, Britain's general practitioners tend to be thoroughly capitalist.

My friend Dr. Badat, for example, has found ways to capitalize on numerous moneymaking opportunities within the National Health Service. With a roster of about four thousand registered patients—more than double the average load for a British family practice—he earns about £90,000 ($125,000) a year on the basic capitation payment from the NHS. He owns the narrow building that houses his surgery and rents it to the NHS for a little more than the monthly mortgage payment. He makes house calls on sick or elderly patients a couple of days each week; this not only brings in extra payments from the NHS but allows him to write off the sleek navy blue Jaguar S-type parked outside the office. Some GPs, particularly in posh neighborhoods, can earn extra income seeing patients privately—patients who are willing to pay $80 or so to avoid a couple of hours in the waiting room. But this option doesn't fly in the working class, multiethnic West London neighborhood where Dr. Badat practices. Until the mid-1990s, Dr. Badat got free vacations, golf clubs, and other lucrative gifts from pharmaceutical companies, but such handouts are now considered bribes and have been banned (both in Britain and in the United States).

The greatest boon to Ahmed Badat, and almost every other British general practitioner, has been an experimental payment called the Index of Quality Indicators. It's an effort to pay for results—to give a doctor more money if he treats his patients successfully and keeps them healthy. The NHS "quality" system is the world's most extensive manifestation of a concept that has become a holy grail for health care managers around the world: pay for performance. This is supposed to replace the standard fee-for-service structure, in which the doctor gets a set fee for a particular treatment, whether the patient gets better or not. In the British version of pay for performance, doctors are graded on about five dozen "quality indicators." The problem with this brilliant idea has been that nobody can agree on the appropriate "quality indicators" to measure a doctor's performance.

In Britain, the gap was filled by the British Medical Association, which established a series of "best practices" for doctors treating specific diseases. The NHS agrees to pay doctors a bonus for carrying out best practices, up to a maximum of about $125,000 per year. This has proven to be an unmitigated gold mine for British doctors. "Most of the stuff in those 'best practices,' I always did it anyway," Dr. Badat told me. "Checking the extremities of patients with diabetes. Getting my hypertensives to take their blood pressure every day. Any doctor would do those things. But now they pay me extra to do it. It's, you know, free money." For example, Dr. Badat has always encouraged his elderly patients to get a flu shot (in Britain, a flu "jab") each autumn; the NHS provides the vaccine for free. Under the quality indicators system, he gets an additional $6 for each shot, as pay for performance. No wonder his nurses wear that red pin saying, ASK ME ABOUT A FREE FLU JAB. Overall, pay for performance has roughly doubled his annual income, to about £210,000 ($296,000) per year.

That income would put Dr. Badat in the top rank of general practitioners in the United States. And a British doctor making that much would come out well ahead of his American counterpart. Dr. Badat pays $4,200 per year for malpractice insurance, about as much as an

American GP might pay in a month. If he were to be sued for mal-practice, he would have a fairly simple means to stop the legal action before it got anywhere. In British law, any doctor who can show that he was following the guidelines approved by NICE for a particular treatment or procedure is immune from a malpractice claim. The result is that doctors in the UK spend much less for malpractice insurance than their peers in the United States and are less inclined to practice "defensive medicine" to avoid a lawsuit. Beyond that, British doctors generally graduate from medical school with little or no debt to pay off, partly because tuition fees are low (about $4,000 per year) and partly because many local governments pay the tuition for medical students from their community.

The reliance on capitation payments—in essence, paying a doctor for keeping his patients healthy—and the broad range of pay-for-performance measures reflect another essential feature of the National Health Service: the system's powerful commitment to preventive med-icine. In a nation where the health system has to care for everybody, sick or well, from cradle to grave, there is a clear incentive to keep people well. The Brits have made a huge bet that it is worth spending money to keep people healthy in the first place, so they don't have to go to the doctor and incur costs for the system. In essence, Britain's NHS has forcefully embraced the old nostrum "An ounce of preven-tion is worth a pound of cure." In chapter 11 we'll consider whether that familiar slogan is true.

EIGHT

Canada: "Sorry to Keep You Waiting"

ON A MAKESHIFT FOOTBALL PITCH IN A SUBURB OF GLAS-gow, a wee slip of a Scots lad took a tumble and banged his knee badly on a rock. It was a painful injury that would leave the boy limping and handicapped for years, but most Canadians would say it was a lucky fall. Many years later, that injury would inspire the universal health care system that has become the pride of Canada and has served as a model for the public financing of health care in several other countries—including the rich, powerful country just south of the border.

For Canadian schoolchildren, the story of Tommy Douglas and his banged-up knee has the legendary quality of George Washington and the cherry tree. But the Tommy Douglas legend has the added virtue of being essentially true. Thomas Clement Douglas was six years old in 1910 when he suffered that injury in Falkirk, Scotland. The boy was still limping, and sometimes using crutches, when his family emigrated to western Canada a year later. Surgery was indicated, but surgery in those days was a luxury for people who had far more money than the struggling Douglas family. By sheer chance, a professor of orthopedics in Winnepeg chose Tommy to be the subject of a demonstration of surgical technique. The operation was a complete success; the boy could walk normally again. But young Tommy was bothered by the unfairness of it: Why was his cure a matter of sheer chance? And why should he get medical care when countless others had no access to treatment?[1]

"I felt that no boy should have to depend either for his leg or his life upon the ability of parents to raise enough money," Douglas wrote in his memoir. "I came to believe that people should be able to get . . . health services irrespective of their individual capacity to pay."[2] When he was elected premier (that is, governor) of the province of Saskatchewan in 1944, Douglas turned that passionate belief into a government-run, single-payer health care system for all of Saskatchewan's 1 million residents. The program was so successful and so popular that residents of other provinces began demanding the same program. The federal government in Ottawa signed on; by 1961 everyone in Canada was covered by a taxpayer-funded hospital insurance program. Today the public health insurance system covers all medical and psychiatric care, in or out of the hospital.

The National Health Insurance model that Tommy Douglas pioneered on the prairies of Saskatchewan has spread around the world. As we'll see in chapter 10, the Asian nation of Taiwan undertook a comprehensive study of developed nations' health care systems and decided to follow the Canadian model. South Korea made the same decision. In 1965, when the U.S. Congress decided to guarantee health care to any American over sixty-five, the Americans adopted both the National Health Insurance model—that is, private providers and public financing—and the name that Tommy Douglas gave it, Medicare.

As it approaches its fiftieth birthday, Canada's universal-coverage system is still a source of national pride, but it is also a matter of national concern. Canadian health care today is not particularly healthy; it is limping along like a poor boy with a broken knee.

The system still records high levels of satisfaction. "The health care system is consistently Canada's most popular social program, and the country's health insurance system is often cited as a defining feature of Canada," an international report noted in 2000.[3] The fact that anybody who needs health care can get it, without payment, satisfies the basic collectivist spirit of the nation. No Canadian dies because he can't afford a doctor; no Canadian goes bankrupt from medical bills. "It's not really part of the Canadian psyche to feel superior to anybody," Marcus Davies, an official with a Canadian medical society, told me. "But there are two areas where we enjoy feeling smugly superior to the United States: hockey and health care." This is mainly because Canada guarantees health care to everyone who needs it while the richer country to the south does not. Beyond that, Canada has better health statistics overall than the United States, a longer healthy life expectancy, and a lower rate of infant mortality. And it achieves all that for about half the cost per capita of the U.S. system. "Canada's cost advantage," the Canadian health care economist Robert Evans, told me, "is due to a much more efficient payment system and to the sheer clout that a universal system has in price negotiations."

Still, the federal and provincial governments have not been willing, or able, to provide the funding Medicare needs. In 2007, Canada spent about 10 percent of GDP on health care, far below the U.S. rate. With that level of spending, it can't keep up with the rapidly rising cost of medicine. The result is a health care system that is "underdoctored," as the Canadians put it. Since the system is in a constant state of scrimping and saving, medicine is a less desirable profession in Canada than it once was; fewer Canadian college students want to become nurses or physicians. To make a bad situation even worse, an official commission in 1991 recommended that Canada reduce the number of students at its medical schools. By the early twenty-first century, when that policy shift bore fruit, the ratio of doctors to patients had fallen across Canada, particularly in rural areas. Today, Canada is trying to graduate more homegrown doctors and import others from the developing world. But the system remains significantly "underdoctored," and it's not clear that government is willing to spend the money to solve that problem.

For acute illness, accident, and emergency care, Canada's system does guarantee that rich or poor can always get the care they need, generally at no cost. But if your medical problem is not urgent enough to require immediate treatment, Canada will almost always keep you waiting.

That was precisely what happened with my bum shoulder. Canada was the only country on my global quest where the waiting list was so long that I never had a chance even to meet an orthopedist or a physical therapist. When I explained my shoulder problem to Dr. Steven Goluboff, a sympathetic general practitioner in Saskatoon, he agreed that I needed a specialist's care. "I can give you a referral to an orthopod," the doctor said. "But the frustrating thing is, it will take ten to twelve months before you can get an appointment." "You mean, I'd have to wait a year to get my shoulder treated?" I asked. "Oh, I'm not talking about treatment," Dr. Goluboff replied. "It will take a year for you to get a consultation. If the orthopedist decides you need surgery, you'll have to wait another six months, eight months, to get that on the schedule."

The waiting periods vary from province to province, and they vary according to the treatment you're waiting for. Orthopedic surgery is notorious for long waiting lines across Canada; other backed-up procedures include MRI scans, cataract surgery, coronary bypass, and radiation treatments for cancer. It has been widely reported, on both sides of the border, that millions of Canadians stuck on the waiting list travel to the United States to pay for the care they could not get in the free Canadian system. This "fact" is satisfying to advocates of private-market health care, both in Canada and in the United States; it seems to prove that government-run health care can't work. In fact, though, the race to the south is mainly fictional. The anecdotal reports are not supported by any statistical research. Expert studies of the "health care refugee" issue have concluded that the actual number of snowbirds heading south for health care is tiny.[4] Canadian officials argue, in fact, that the number of Americans who come north for drugs or treatment is greater than the number of Canadians heading south. Rather, most Canadians deal with the waiting list by waiting. Statistics suggest that those who need care urgently can get it. But anybody whose problem can wait will wait, somewhat mollified by the awareness that everybody else is waiting, too. "Canadians don't mind the waiting list so much," observes the Princeton economist Uwe Reinhardt, who grew up in Canada, "so long as the rich Canadian and the poor Canadian have to wait about the same amount of time."

WHEN TOMMY DOUGLAS'S Scottish family settled in Canada shortly before World War I, the rich Canadian had access to medical care and the poor Canadian did not, except at a few widely scattered public clinics. The Douglas family was in the latter category; whatever medical care they received was due either to charity or to the lucky happenstance of a professor who needed to demonstrate knee surgery. Tommy himself helped sustain the family, working as a messenger, a retail clerk, and a prizefighter. As final proof that the knee was fully cured, he won the Manitoba Lightweight Championship in 1922. He became a printer's assistant, a job that required membership in the International Typographical Union. That introduced him to the world of organized labor and its politics. Through his progressive contacts, Douglas came into the ken of J. S. Woodsworth, a Methodist minister and a fiery populist who preached the "social gospel," the idea that the church must be concerned not only about the next world but also about injustice and inequality in this one. In 1924 Douglas began studying for the ministry, and in 1930 he landed a job as pastor of a rural Baptist church in Weyburn, across the border from Winnipeg, in the province of Saskatchewan.

The years of the Great Depression and the long drought are known in western Canada as the Dirty Thirties, a time when the farmers of the prairie provinces had no crop, no money, no food, and of course, no medical care. For the young pastor in Weyburn, the utter lack of health care for the sick was particularly difficult to bear: "Out in the country I performed funeral services," Douglas wrote years later. "I buried [two] young men in their thirties, who died because there was no doctor readily available, and they hadn't the money to get proper care. They were buried in coffins made by the local people out of ordinary board. The smell permeated the church."[5]

Gradually, the Reverend T. C. Douglas came to believe that charity would never be enough to help the endless lines of desperate people. He decided that government control of production, markets, and social services was the only way to distribute wealth fairly. In the early 1930s, Douglas joined a populist party—the Co-operative Commonwealth Federation—that hoped to turn Saskatchewan into a cooperative socialist commonwealth. As a CCF candidate, he became a popular stump politician throughout the province, a charming raconteur who had a funny story for every occasion. At the start of one speech, he complained that he had to spend a lot his time answering false charges from the centrist parties about the CCF. "People ask if it's true that we're going to close the churches," Tommy said in his genial way. "I answer, 'Certainly not.' They ask if it's true that we are going to take away people's farms. I answer, 'Certainly not.' Once, a woman with five or six children scampering around her legs asked, 'Is it true you're going to take away our children?' I answered, 'Certainly not.' She said, 'I thought it was too good to be true.'"[6]

In 1944, Douglas was the CCF candidate for premier of the province, declaring forthrightly that he intended to head "the first socialist government in North America." In his speeches, he always brought up his youthful knee injury and promised voters that he would create a universal hospital insurance program so that nobody in the province would have to rely on the whims of chance, as he had, to get necessary medical care. Almost everybody in Canada was familiar with the famous Beveridge Report in Great Britain, so the idea of government-run, tax-financed health care was not seen as wacky or impractical. Indeed, the promise of free health care for all was a key reason that Douglas won the election.

Once in office, Tommy Douglas called in a famous medical historian, Henry Sigerist, of Johns Hopkins Medical School, to design a course toward universal coverage. Sigerist recommended that the province move toward "socialized medicine"—his term for government payment of medical bills from private providers—but do so gradually, starting with maternity patients, the elderly, etc. Douglas, true to form, ignored the "gradually" part. His administration started building new hospitals all over the province and set up a provincial insurance plan to pay everybody's hospital bills. On January 1, 1947, hospital care became free at the point of service for every resident of Saskatchewan.

The system worked. Partly because many new doctors were moving to the province, partly because postwar hunger for Saskatchewan's wheat crop helped fill the provincial treasury, there proved to be enough capacity and money to meet the soaring increase in medical demand. Government-funded medicine was so popular that Tommy Douglas, the head of a radical minority party, remained premier through five elections. Beyond its success in Saskatchewan, the Douglas hospital insurance plan had a powerful "demonstration effect" across Canada: If it could work in Saskatchewan, other provinces decided they could make it work as well. The hospital insurance system was eventually adopted in every province and territory.

But Tommy Douglas had broader ambitions. Running for his fifth term in 1960, he promised a tax-funded public insurance plan that would cover all medical treatment, in or out of the hospital. Having won reelection on this pledge, Douglas gave birth in 1961 to a system he called Medicare, permitting everybody to go to any doctor without getting a bill. It was not an easy delivery. The doctors—many of whom had emigrated to Saskatchewan from Britain specifically to escape government-run medicine—were bitterly opposed. On the day the plan went into effect, in July 1962, virtually every physician in the province went on strike, refusing to treat anything but acute emergency cases. Douglas, of course, fired back with both barrels—the Saskatchewan Medical Society, he said, was "abominable, despicable, and scurrilous"—and the public sided strongly with the new Medicare plan. After twenty-three days, the doctors folded, and once again all of Canada watched carefully to see if Saskatchewan's universal health insurance scheme would succeed.

In practice, Medicare proved to be both affordable and popular in Saskatchewan, and the "demonstration effect" was again powerful. Under intense public pressure, the federal government created a Royal Commission to study a national system based on the Saskatchewan model. The group was chaired by Supreme Court Justice Emmett Hall, a pro-business conservative who would seem to have almost nothing in common with an unabashed socialist like Tommy Douglas. But when Hall issued his report in 1964, it sounded like one of Douglas's tub-thumping populist sermons. "Economic growth is not the sole aim of our society," the Hall Report said. "The value of a human life must be decided without regard to . . . economic considerations. We must take into account the human and spiritual aspects involved." With that establishment stamp of approval, the drive for a national Medicare system proved unstoppable. A bill to establish Saskatchewan-style health care on a national basis passed unanimously in both houses of Parliament. With financial support and guidance from Ottawa, every province and territory set up its own Medicare plan, paying the bills for all medical, psychiatric, and hospital care.

By the 1980s, tough, determined Tommy Douglas needed help from Medicare himself. At the age of seventy-four, too deaf to hear traffic noises, he walked into the street right in front of a bus; from his hospital bed, the former boxing champion conceded that he was badly injured but added, "If you think I'm in bad shape, you should see the bus." By the time Douglas died, in 1986, his health care plan was a central and cherished aspect of Canadian life. Today, Saskatchewan's Medicare network is supervised from the headquarters of the health ministry in Regina, an imposing edifice known as the T. C. Douglas Building. When the Canadian Broadcasting Corporation polled the nation in 2004 to choose "the greatest Canadian of all time," Tommy Douglas won by a landslide, easily beating out the likes of Alexander Graham Bell and Wayne Gretzky.[7]

CANADA'S GOVERNMENT-FINANCED Medicare program is sometimes called a single-payer system, but this is technically inaccurate. Because of its long history of decentralized government, Canada really has a thirteen-payer system. Each of the ten provinces and three territories operates its own Medicare plan, with some difference in fee structures and rules. Some provinces pay 100 percent of every doctor and hospital bill; others require patients to make a co-pay or pay a deductible before the government insurance kicks in. Still, Canadian Medicare is a closely coordinated structure that works like a single-payer system in many ways, because the federal government provides much of the funding and sets many of the rules for the individual provincial plans. That gives Medicare serious clout when it comes to negotiating fees and prices for treatment, medical equipment, and drugs. Among other savings, Canadians pay one-quarter to one-half the price Americans do for the same pill made by the same drug company; that's why a flourishing cross-border trade in drugs developed, with Americans going north to fill their prescriptions at the cheaper Canadian prices.

The governing document that establishes the basic framework of Medicare is the Canada Health Act of 1984, a national law that makes the rules each provincial plan has to follow in order to receive financial aid from the federal government. In theory, these rules are simply advisory, but since no province can afford to do without the federal subsidy, the act is effectively mandatory. The law sets forth five basic principles that each provincial plan must follow. They are principles that would make sense for any national health plan relying on government financing:

1. **Public Administration.** Each province's health insurance system must by operated by a public body on a not-for-profit basis.
2. **Comprehensiveness.** Each plan must pay for all "medically necessary" services. The definition of "necessary" tends to change over time, with new treatments and drugs regularly added to the list.
3. **Universality.** Every resident of the province must have the same access as everybody else to treatments and drugs covered by the plan.
4. **Portability.** The provincial plan has to pay for coverage anywhere in the country (and, often, in foreign countries).
5. **Accessibility.** Doctors must treat everybody for the same fee, regardless of age or illness.

In practice, the Canada Health Act means that access to care is largely uniform across the country, despite some province-by-province variation. Most Canadians pay nothing for a doctor visit, nothing for the emergency room, nothing for a hospital stay, nothing for an MRI scan or other diagnostic test, nothing for an injection or a vaccination. Mental health care is commonly part of the package (although you may wait months to see a psychiatrist). Normal dental care is not covered, but dental surgery performed in a hospital is free. Most provinces pay for ambulance services. Although prescriptions are cheaper than in the United States, people in most provinces have to pay for their drugs; Medicare picks up the drug bill for the poor, the elderly, and people with chronic illness who need constant medication. Canadians are required to pay out of pocket for Viagra, on the grounds that the public system should not finance "lifestyle" drugs; but Medicare does cover the cost of the AIDS cocktail of drugs for those who need it.

In other words, most medical costs in Canada are covered by the government health insurance plan. And yet most Canadians—roughly two out of three working people—also have private health insurance to pay the tab for things that aren't covered by the system, like dental care, private hospital rooms, prescriptions, childbirth classes, and so on. You can't use private insurance to cut to the front of the waiting line, but you can buy things the public system doesn't offer. At City Hospital in Saskatoon, a dramatically modern white building that looks like a fancy private hospital in some upscale U.S. suburb, new mothers pay nothing for childbirth and hospitalization if they stay in a standard maternity ward with four other new mothers and their babies. But the hospital also boasts the Queen Victoria Room, a much larger private room with leather couches and a large-screen plasma TV. That room costs $150 per night; mothers with the right kind of private insurance can stay there and bill the insurance company. Since all major procedures in Canada are covered by Medicare, the supplemental insurance plans generally don't have to pay any huge bills. Accordingly, private insurance is cheap in Canada—so cheap that many employers provide it as a free fringe benefit.

Even though private health insurance plays a supplemental and decidedly minor role in Canadian health care, its very existence is the source of considerable angst in medical and political circles. The constant fear is that rich people will turn more and more to private insurance and away from Medicare. The result would be "two-tier medicine," a term that is as pejorative in Canada as "socialized medicine" is in the United States. Many fear that if Canada did move to two-tier medicine, the rich might get better care, with less waiting, than the poor. The rich getting better access to health care—that's a fact of life that we take for granted in the United States. But in Canada, such a result would violate the powerful egalitarian impulse that is a crucial element of the national culture.

To avoid this threat, all provinces make it illegal for patients, or insurance plans, to pay privately for any medical service that is covered by the Medicare system. If you want Viagra or Botox treatment or a circumcision for your baby, private insurance can cover those procedures, because the public system won't pay for them. But the private plans can't pay for a flu shot or a cardiac bypass or a total shoulder arthroplasty, because those procedures are provided to everyone by Medicare. Beyond that, it is virtually impossible to find private care in most of the country. A doctor or hospital that bills Medicare is not allowed to practice privately as well or bill patients directly. Since virtually every doctor in Canada relies on Medicare for his income, very few offer private treatment.

That makes for a thoroughly egalitarian system, but there's one major problem: A lot of medical care that people would be willing to pay for, if they were allowed to pay, is hard to get under Medicare. The issue is waiting lists. Yes, Canada's Medicare system will replace my aching shoulder for free—but only if I wait a year for a consultation with an orthopedic specialist, then wait another six months or so to get a spot in the operating room. If my shoulder really hurts, I may not want to wait eighteen months for the public system to get around to me. But under the law, I have no choice. Even if I have enough money or private insurance coverage, I can't buy immediate care. Some argue that the ban on paying privately for a given procedure is tantamount to a ban on that procedure altogether—that access to a waiting list is not the same thing as access to treatment.

This argument came to a head in a blockbuster Canadian Supreme Court decision, a ruling that could threaten the very foundations of Medicare. A sixty-seven-year-old citizen of Quebec was suffering from a painful hip condition; his physician, Dr. Jacques Chaoulli, recommended hip-replacement surgery. But that recommendation gave the patient nothing more than a place on the waiting list. After nine months had passed, Dr. Chaoulli went to court on behalf of his patient. He argued that a nine-month wait for an elderly man in severe pain amounted to denial of the right to medical care; thus the patient should be allowed to get the operation privately and bill his insurance company for the cost. To the astonishment of just about everybody, the Supreme Court agreed. "The prohibition on obtaining private health insurance," said the court's opinion in *Chaoulli* v. *Quebec*, "while it might be constitutional in circumstances where health care services are reasonable as to both quality and timeliness, is not constitutional where the public system fails to deliver reasonable services."[8]

The Chaoulli decision came down in 2005, and many predicted that it would lead quickly to the dreaded two-tier medicine. That may eventually be the result, but so far it has not happened. Instead, the decision has jolted governments into providing more, and faster, care. The federal government and the provinces have agreed to spend more money, bring in more doctors, and reduce the waiting lists. "We're not going to have a two-tier health care system in this country," Prime Minister Paul Martin said after the decision. "What we want to do is to strengthen the public health care system." Quebec's provincial government responded to the Chaoulli case by setting specific time limits for the completion of hip-replacement and many other procedures. If nothing else, the decision seems to have spurred a new round of spending on health care across Canada. But the fact remains that doctor shortages and waiting lists continue to be a basic frustration for anybody who has to rely on Canada's health care system.

"IT'S SO REWARDING, and *soooo* frustrating, to work in this system," Dr. Steven Goluboff said to me, smiling at a baby girl he had delivered a day before. "It is rewarding to provide anybody the medical care they need, without worrying about bills or paperwork or malpractice problems. But it's so frustrating, just the day-to-day frustration of the waiting lists. If my patient needs an MRI or a psychiatric evaluation or shoulder surgery, all I can do is put her on the list and tell her to wait. It could be months. It could be a year. That's kind of"—here he stopped for a minute to choose the right adjective—"kind of . . . scandalous, is what it is, that people have to wait so long for the treatment they need."

Dr. Goluboff, an energetic sixty-year-old bantam with a balding pate and a light gray beard, has no doubt that running a family practice in the heart of Saskatoon, Saskatchewan, is exactly what he wants to do. The son of a doctor—his dad, in fact, was one of those who struck against Tommy Douglas's Medicare plan in 1961—Goluboff always knew what his life's work would be. As a child, he dressed up as a doctor on Halloween. As an adult, he routinely sees fifty or more patients per day—and that's after his morning rounds at the city's three hospitals and a few early surgical procedures, such as vasectomies and circumcisions.

Goluboff works in a cramped corner office across the street from Saskatoon City Hospital. The walls are adorned with his diploma, the plaque he won for being named Family Physician of the Year, and a poster that sets forth ONE HUNDRED WAYS TO LIVE TO ONE HUNDRED. Tip #100, in bold print: LISTEN TO YOUR DOCTOR. The office has a chart listing the prices of procedures not covered by the Medicare system: circumcision, $100; IUD, $100; cautery of warts, $40. The bookshelves are stacked high with boxes of drug samples Goluboff has received from pharmaceutical salesmen: Robaxacet, Uremol HC, Nasonex, Detrol. "If a patient doesn't have a [private insurance] plan, paying for prescriptions is tough," the doctor says. "The more I can give them for free, the more likely they are to get the medicine they need."

Like almost every doctor in almost every country, Goluboff complains that he isn't paid enough for his hard work; in fact, his income is about half as much as an American family doctor might expect to earn. Still, he drives a BMW convertible and belongs to the town's leading country club. And Canada's system gives him certain advantages that American doctors would envy. He carries malpractice insurance but has no idea how much it costs, because the provincial government pays the premium for him. His office has no file cases full of patient records, because Canada's coordinated system has made all medical records digital. He never has to deal with money. Patients pay nothing to see him; the provincial Medicare office pays all his fees at the end of each month. The tuition costs for a medical degree run about half what they would be at a public university in the United States, so Canadian doctors start their careers with far less debt than their counterparts south of the border.

For an American observer sitting in the corner of the office, the striking thing about Steven Goluboff's practice was the broad socio-economic range of his patients. There were middle-class mothers bringing the kids in for vaccinations and well-dressed businesspeople complaining of headaches or asthma—just what you'd expect to see in a family doctor's office in the United States. But there were also un-washed, ragged patients who didn't appear to have a dime to their name—people you probably wouldn't find in a typical U.S. doctor's office. But they had no problem seeing a doctor in Canada when they needed it.

One thirtysomething woman, pierced and tattooed and smelling vividly of perspiration and tobacco, told the doctor that she had been living "pretty much on the street" after her boyfriend threw her out for drinking too much. She had no job, no money. She hadn't been to a doctor in years. But she was feeling "kind of punk," she said; she didn't feel like eating; her side ached. Dr. Goluboff extended his hand and gently pressed the right side of her abdomen; the woman jumped back, wincing with pain. Within seconds, Goluboff was on the phone to the emergency ward. "I think we've got an acute appy here," he said. "I'll put her in an ambulance and get her over there in twenty minutes." Now the woman was worried: "Hospital? Ambulance? Do they expect me to pay for that?" "No," the doctor replied, "you don't have to pay for anything. We're going to fix you up—probably remove your appendix, which you don't need anyway. And of course, we're not going to charge you for it."

Moments like that make the daily struggle worthwhile for any doctor. "There's a good chance we saved a life there," Dr. Goluboff told me later. "And it's only because she knew she could come in to see me for free when she felt 'kind of punk.' Acute cases like that—that's where Canadian medicine really shines. And anybody in this country will get that kind of care. But it's *sooooo* frustrating that other people, nonacute cases, just go on a waiting list. Somebody told me that I should have the words 'Sorry to keep you waiting' carved on my gravestone, because that's what I'm always telling patients."

CAN WE LEARN ANYTHING about health care from our closest English-speaking neighbor? As we've seen in other countries, Canada's experience teaches us that it is possible to provide medical care for everybody—and still spend far less per person than the United States does now—if a country decides that it has a moral obligation to make health care universal. Canada shows again that a coordinated system of payment (whether it's single-payer or thirteen-payer) has enough negotiating clout with health care providers to get serious control over costs. But even with that market power, Canada demonstrates that health care costs are rising fast just about everywhere. A system like Canada's Medicare, which tries to stint on expenditures, is going to face the kind of frustrating waiting lists that plague Canadian medicine.

The most distinctive lesson we could take, though, from Canada's health care system is the key point of the Tommy Douglas saga: Universal health care coverage doesn't have to start at the national level. Once Douglas established free hospital care in a poor rural province and made it work, the demonstration effect drove other provinces to do the same thing. And once Douglas established his taxpayer-funded Medicare system to pay all medical bills in the province, the demonstration effect quickly turned Saskatchewan's idea into a national health care system that covers everybody.

If one of our fifty states were to try the same thing and make it work, the demonstration effect could spread across the United States. And if that were to happen, it would bear out one of Tommy Douglas's most famous predictions: "If people see that we can provide health care to all, free at the point of service, so that any person, rich or poor, can get the medical treatment he needs—if people elsewhere see that, they'll want it, too."

NINE

Out of Pocket

MRS. RAMA CAME SWEEPING INTO MY HOSPITAL ROOM THE second time wearing an off-white sari with pale green piping, trailed again by the retinue of assistants and interpreters we met in the first chapter of this book. It was a couple of days after our original meeting, and she had completed her yajnopathic analysis of my place in the cosmos. As she sat on the floor of my hospital room, moving the rocks and shells and statuettes around her wooden board, she solemnly informed me of the good news: The stars were properly aligned for me to be healed. Thus my treatment could begin at the Arya Vaidya Chikitsalayam, India's leading center of the traditional medicine called Ayurveda. As usual, Mrs. Rama was the epitome of unruffled self-assurance. "The star charts leave no doubt," she told me with complete confidence. "Your sore shoulder will definitely improve during your treatment here."

With that, my medical care was entrusted to the *vaidyas,* or physicians, at the famous clinic. I embarked on a treatment regimen that involved prayers to the Hindu god of healing, meditation on the sacred text Bhagavad Gita, an endless round of herbal oils and ointments and medications, and a daily dose of manipulation and massage conducted in strict accordance with instructions left by the ancient sages of yoga.

The treatment and the medications I received at the *chikitsalayam* clearly reflected traditional Indian medicine. But while my treatment was traditional, it was not typical. That is an important distinction for this book. Under the health care systems—or, more precisely, nonsystems—of India and most poor countries, getting any form of medical care is not "typical."

In much of Africa, South America, and South Asia, the "health care system" is brutally simple: The rich, the military, and sometimes other government employees get medical care; everybody else stays sick or dies. In countries where almost all resources are needed to provide food, water, and shelter, medical care is a luxury, and a scarce one at that. As we saw earlier, rich nations spend a significant share of their gross national product on health care—about 17 percent in the United States, 11 percent in Switzerland, 8 percent in Japan. In Nigeria, in contrast, total medical spending amounts to less than 1 percent of GDP; the country spends $5 per person per year on health care. Some nations spend less than that. In most African countries, the bulk of public spending on health care, whether the funds are domestic or foreign aid, is aimed at the lethal epidemic of HIV-AIDS. There is little or nothing left over to pay for treatment of all other diseases or accidents. Thus people have to pay for treatment themselves—and if they can't pay, there's no treatment, unless the patient is lucky enough to have access to doctors from an international charity organization.

In India, as in other "developing nations"—a standard term nowadays for the world's poorer countries—it is not at all normal for most people to see a doctor or to receive any kind of structured medical treatment. Of India's 1.1 billion people, about 750 million live in rural villages; most of those villagers never see a doctor or a hospital. A woman in childbirth, with luck, might have the services of a local midwife who has learned traditional techniques from earlier generations of midwives. A person with a snakebite or a broken bone or an abscessed tooth may have access to a local healer, who might use traditional herbal medicines, or perhaps yajnopathy, to attempt a cure. In a tiny Tamil Nadu village called Telungupalayam, I met a doctor— he had no formal training, but he was considered to be a doctor of medicine—named Arjunan. He was famous across southern India as a healer of polio. That bone-twisting disease, which was wiped out decades ago in the West, still cripples children in southern India, where the Salk and Sabin vaccines are not widely available. Arjunan treats polio cases by encasing children's legs in large vats of sand or lashing their limbs to poles. They live like that in his hospital—a crumbling concrete structure with rough cement floors and windows without glass—for weeks at a time. At first glance, the hospital looked like a torture chamber. But the children I met, standing straight up with their legs buried in sand, seemed grateful to get the treatment. Frequently, a parent or relative moves into the hospital with the child to provide companionship and serve meals. After long periods of immobilization, Arjunan told me, the children's legs and backs begin to straighten. His hospital was full of before-and-after photos that seemed to show significant improvement in his young patients. I asked Dr. Arjunan where he had learned this technique. His "medical school," he said, was his home; his professors were his grandfather and father, who taught him techniques passed down from their grandfathers. Arjunan said he receives some support from the national health ministry in New Delhi, and he also asks his patients' families to pay what they can, out of pocket.

When health care economists describe the basic models of health care systems—the Bismarck Model, the Beveridge Model, etc.—a standard term to describe the systems, or nonsystems, in poor countries is the Out-of-Pocket Model. Since there is little or no government money to pay for health care and there is no health insurance, most medical treatment must be paid for by the patient. If a sick person has some money, he pays in currency. If there's no money, the patient pays in potatoes or pottery or dairy products or babysitting services or whatever he can scratch up. In the Solu-Khumbu region of northern Nepal, I visited the Amji Clinic. It was a simple rectangular building of rough plaster, and each of the walls was a different color. Dr. Sherab Tenzin, who runs the place, explained that patients sometimes offered to pay for their care by painting the hospital, and different patients happened to arrive with different colors of paint. Dr. Tenzin lets them paint away. "It provides some dignity to pay for the service they receive," he explained.

The World Health Organization tracks almost every imaginable kind of data about health care around the world, and one of the numbers it records is the percentage of health care spending in each nation that comes from the patients' pockets. This percentage tends to be small in the rich, industrialized countries that have health insurance systems, whether public or private. In the world's poorer countries—the Out-of-Pocket countries—the percentage of out-of-pocket payments tends to be much higher. The table on the following page provides a sample.

Some poor countries report out-of-pocket spending below 50 percent, for example, Tanzania (39.3 percent) and Kenya (35.9 percent). In these countries, the government pays for more than half of all health care spending, often channeling funds received from foreign-aid programs or international charities. But this government spending is generally not evenly distributed. A standard pattern among poorer countries is that nearly all the money spent on health care is spent in the national capital; wealthy people and government employees, who mainly live in the capital city, are just about the only people who have regular access to a doctor or a hospital. So that's where the health care spending is focused. In rural Kenya, almost no money is spent on health

OUT-OF-POCKET HEALTH SPENDING, 2001

Country	% of total health spending
Myanmar	82.2
India	82.1
Nigeria	76.8
Pakistan	75.6
Egypt	73.0
Cambodia	72.0
Indonesia	68.7
Yemen	65.0
China	59.9
Armenia	58.8
Mexico	51.4
. . .	
USA	14.7
UK	3.1

Source: WHO, World Health Report, 2003.

care, because there are almost no doctors or hospitals to provide the care. In Ethiopia, the WHO says, only 20 percent of the population—almost all of them residents of the capital, Addis Ababa—have access to any medical care at all.[1]

The Out-of-Pocket payment system also applies to drugs, which means that most people in the developing nations don't get modern medications. The World Health Organization says that 67 percent of the world's population has no "regular" access to drugs.[2] That means that if you get sick, the nearest clinic or hospital may or may not have a stock of the pill that could cure you. It's random. And since people paying out of pocket often can't afford medication even if it is available, many die of diseases that could be treated with pills that are on the shelf of the local clinic. To make a tragic situation even more tragic, many poor countries see imported medicine as a source of government revenue: They insist on collecting import duties, port fees, license fees, and so forth on medicines even if the pills have been donated for free by the manufacturer or a charity. In Nigeria, medical charities that donate mosquito netting to protect sleeping children from malaria are routinely required to pay import duties before they can distribute the free, life-saving nets.[3]

The medical implications of the Out-of-Pocket Model are sadly predictable. Because most people can't get treatment or medication, there are millions of deaths each year in Africa, south Asia, and Latin America from diseases that have disappeared in the developed world: polio, malaria, leprosy, etc. When this pattern of life and death is turned into statistics, it turns out—no surprise here—that countries using the Out-of-Pocket Model of health care have the world's shortest life expectancy. Among the wealthy nations, life expectancy (averaged among men and women) generally ranges from seventy-five to eighty-one years; in the United States, the average life expectancy at birth is just over seventy-seven years. But look at the average life span in some of the countries where people don't have access to health care (see page 149).

LIFE EXPECTANCY AT BIRTH, 2002

Mozambique	32 years
Zambia	35
Malawi	38
Zimbabwe	40
Afghanistan	47
Cambodia	57
Nepal	59
India	63
Bolivia	64

Source: U.S. Census Bureau, International Data Base:
www.census.gov/ftp/pub/ipc/www/idsum.html.

The absence of health care is not the only reason that the average person dies in his thirties or forties in some of these countries; starvation, harsh living conditions, warfare, HIV-AIDS, and violence all play a role in keeping lives short. But the fact that people rarely, if ever, see a doctor is a key factor. Simply put, an out-of-pocket health care system lets large numbers of people die from illnesses or trauma that could be treated.

This pattern also holds in the only wealthy country that uses the Out-of-Pocket Model for a significant portion of the population: the United States. Most Americans are covered by health insurance, Medicare, or Medicaid and can get medical treatment; at any given time, though, more than 40 million residents who are too young for Medicare and too well-off for Medicaid go without health insurance. For these people, medical care is mainly an out-of-pocket thing. It's true that Americans who are acutely ill can go to a hospital emergency ward and receive treatment, whether they are insured or not. But that option applies only to people in active labor or on the verge of death; otherwise, the uninsured have to pay for their care—and, often, can't afford to. The impact on health is clear. Many studies show that uninsured Americans are more likely to get sick and stay sick longer than their neighbors with health insurance. A U.S. government study found that accident victims who are uninsured are 37 percent more likely to die from their injuries than somebody with insurance.[4] As we noted at the beginning of this book, government and academic studies report that more than twenty thousand Americans die each year from treatable diseases, because they don't have health insurance and can't afford to pay for treatment out of pocket. Beyond that, Americans on the Out-of-Pocket Model generally don't get early diagnosis of potentially fatal diseases—cancer, hypertension, diabetes—and thus are more likely to suffer and die from these ailments.

It's no surprise that a nation's overall health status almost always reflects its overall wealth. The people who live in rich countries tend to have good health and longer lives. If you make a graph that compares personal income to life expectancy in all the nations of the world, the two lines on the chart go up together almost in lockstep; the higher the GDP per capita, the longer people live. The biggest exception to this rule—the obvious outlier on that chart—is Cuba.

The island nation of 11 million that the Castro brothers have run as a totalitarian Communist fiefdom for more than forty years is one of the poorer nations in Latin America. It has a per-capita income of around $4,000 per year; its housing stock is mainly wooden hovels where electricity and hot water are iffy propositions; its farmers tend their sugarcane fields in battered, forty-year-old Soviet tractors held together with wire and duct tape. And yet Cuban health statistics are on par with the best in the world. Life expectancy at birth, according to the World Health Organization, is longer than seventy-seven years—about the same as in rich nations with six times as much per capita income.[5] Infant mortality rates are actually lower than in the United States. Cuba spends about 6 percent of its GDP on health care, a lower proportion than almost any wealthy country but considerably higher than other poor nations.

Unlike most other poor countries, Cuba has a health care system that provides universal coverage, with no out-of-pocket expenditure. (Officially, at least. An American physician who had taught in Cuba told me that people do sometimes offer a doctor cash as a way to jump to the head of the waiting line.) Of the systems described in this book, Cuba's is closest to the Beveridge Model, although the inspiration for Cuba was not Britain but, rather, the state-run hospital system in the Soviet Union, Castro's first benefactor. In the Cuban system, all hospitals are government-owned, almost all doctors and dentists are government employees, and all the bills are paid by government, through general taxation. The Cuban Constitution declares that every citizen has "a right to health protection and care," and the government says it has stationed a doctor and nurse in every rural village. Most countries wouldn't have the manpower to do that, but Cuba has more doctors and nurses per capita than any other nation, according to the WHO. Its medical schools train doctors from all over the world (including several dozen American students studying for an M.D., tuition free, at the Escuela Latinoamericana de Ciencias Médicas, just north of Havana). Under a policy called Medical Diplomacy, the Castros not only provide free medical education for foreign students but also export trained doctors to Venezuela, Bolivia, and other Latin American states. In return, those countries provide the poor island nation with oil and food at cut-rate prices.

In the World Health Organization's ranking of overall health system performance, Cuba came in thirty-ninth, two places below the United States. The WHO gave Cuba high scores for fairness but lower scores for preventive medicine and for its run-down medical facilities. (Of course, fairness and equal treatment extend only so far; when Fidel Castro himself fell ill in 2007, medical experts were flown in from Europe to treat him.)

The Out-of-Pocket Model of health care is generally found in poor countries. As poor countries industrialize and move out of poverty, they often use their new wealth to develop some kind of national health care system that transfers at least some of the financial burden from patients' pockets to government or employers. The rapidly industrializing "new tigers" of Southeast Asia exemplify that trend; as South Korea, Singapore, and Taiwan moved into the ranks of the world's richer nations, they all set up national health care systems to replace out-of-pocket payment. The results can be dramatic, both for the fiscal status of individual citizens and for the health status of the whole population. As we'll see in the next chapter, Taiwan introduced a Canadian-style National Health Insurance system in 1994. The result: Out-of-pocket payments for health care fell from about 75 percent to less than 5 percent.

In short, most nations try to drop the Out-of-Pocket Model as they grow richer. But the world's most populous nation, China, has gone the opposite direction. Since the 1980s, the cadres overseeing China's transformation to a market economy have also transformed health care, from a universal government system to a nonsystem that puts most of the financial burden of health care on the patient. In 1978, when Chairman Mao's "barefoot doctors" were running government-funded clinics in almost every rural community, out-of-pocket payment in China came to 20 percent of health care costs, not much more than in some wealthy nations. By 2005, with medicine mostly privatized, about 60 percent of all health care costs were paid from the patients' pockets, which ranks China with the world's poorest countries. For wealthy people in the big eastern cities, China today has excellent medical care in clean, modern hospitals. But for hundreds of millions of people in the desperately poor rural areas, medicine is an unaffordable luxury. Millions of Chinese die each year because they don't have the money to pay for medical care. Seriously ill Chinese patients sometimes sneak out of the hospital and go home, because they don't want to leave their families with big hospital bills after they die.

When I was traveling the world looking for lessons Americans could benefit from, several economists suggested I look at China as an example of what not to do. "Just to make your American readers feel better," advised Ikegami Naoki, the health care expert at Keio University's hospital in Tokyo, "you ought to tell them about China. It has all the problems of American health care but none of the benefits." "To many in the United States," wrote Harvard professor William Hsiao, "China's portrait of pockets of medical affluence in the midst of declining financial access and exploding costs and inefficiency will sound depressingly familiar."[6] What galls these experts is that China, virtually alone among nations, has gone backward in terms of health care. Mao's Cooperative Medical System was spartan but universal and essentially free—a poor man's version of Britain's Beveridge Model. It produced impressive results: From 1952 to 1982, life expectancy in China increased from thirty-five to sixty-eight years, and many contagious diseases were controlled. In the early 1980s, though, this government-run system essentially shut down, and China reverted to the Out-of-Pocket Model for most of its 1.3 billion people. The results are clear. Infant and child mortality rates actually increased in China during the first decade of the twenty-first century; life expectancy is unchanged since the '80s; some infectious diseases are causing epidemics not seen in decades.[7]

SINCE THE OUT-OF-POCKET COUNTRIES have fewer trained doctors than the richer nations, they tend to rely far more on traditional medicine and methods. For a couple of billion people in the developing world, a village healer—like Arjunan, the Indian practitioner who had his polio patients stand for weeks in vats of sand—maybe the only "doctor" they'll ever see. In some African countries, 80 percent of all medical care is provided by traditional healers. While the poor countries plead with the developed world to supply them with Western doctors and medicine, the West is returning the compliment. In the rich countries—the United States, Europe, and Japan—there has been something of a boom in the fields known as TM (traditional medicine) and CAM (complementary and alternative medicine). The U.S. National Institutes of Health get so many queries about Ayurveda, acupuncture, homeopathy, and so on, that they have set up an office to study these approaches: the National Center for Complementary and Alternative Medicine (or, to use the bureaucratic acronym, NCCAM, pronounced "en-cam").

One of NCCAM's major functions is to run studies to determine whether this alternative stuff works as well as Western-style treatment and Western wonder drugs. At any given time, NCCAM has several dozen double-blind clinical trials up and running. In 2010, the agency had ongoing studies to test the efficacy and safety of such CAM approaches as acupuncture, acupressure, electroacupuncture, ginkgo biloba, milk thistle, mistletoe, naturopathy, tai chi, and yoga.[8] A key reason for these studies is to decide who should pay for alternative treatments. If an American who has a standard health insurance policy uses milk thistle or yoga to deal with an ailment, should the insurance company pay the bill? Generally, the insurance plans restrict their coverage to allopathic medical techniques—that is, the methods and medications taught in Western medical schools. But there has been strong political pressure on the insurers to cover alternative approaches as well: Some state legislatures have mandated that health insurance plans cover acupuncture, massage, and other popular forms of "alternative" treatment. When NCCAM finds—as it often does—that some ancient technique or herbal remedy doesn't work, that conclusion helps the insurance industry resist the pressure to pay. With U.S. medicine already the most expensive in the world, the argument runs, the last thing we need is a legislative mandate to pay for treatment that is useless.

In the poorer nations, of course, there's no argument about this, because there is no insurance system to pay for any medical bills, be they Western or CAM. And so people go to the traditional healer or buy herbal medications or lie down for Ayurvedic massage and just pay out of pocket.

Sometimes there's a conflict between traditional and modern medicine; some countries resist Western doctors and medication in the belief that their local remedies work better (or because Western medicine, particularly for treating HIV-AIDS, is far too expensive for poor countries or patients). The classic case is South Africa, where the government of President Thabo Mbeki insisted for years that traditional medicines made from lemon and beetroot were superior to Western antiretroviral drugs for treating the nation's spreading AIDS epidemic. For the most part, though, people in Asia, Africa, and Latin America take an all-inclusive approach to medicine, looking for the best results, whether traditional or modern.

You can see this dynamic at work in the Solu-Khumbu region of Nepal—it's the stony, almost impassable mountain country at the base of Everest, and the homeland of the Sherpas. The region has a couple of Western medical and dental clinics and a few pharmacies selling Tylenol and other Western medicines. But there are also clinics practicing ancient Tibetan herbal medicine, not to mention the Nepali shamans, or *dhami,* who will chant a prayer or bless an amulet to help a sick person in return for a contribution. When it comes to health care, the Sherpas have no trouble juggling the ancient and the up-to-date.

"People here are absolutely multimedia about medicine," said Heather Culbert, a Canadian M.D. Who was working as a volunteer at the Khunde Clinic, a Canadian-funded Western-style hospital. "They come in here to get vaccinated against flu or polio, because they know that works; and then they walk an hour to get an amulet from the monastery to ward off the same disease. They think that works, too."

In Nepal and other developing countries, the various medical practitioners often work cooperatively. The Amji Clinic—the place with walls of different colors—is in the village of Namche, about an hour's trek from the Canadian clinic at Khunde. Dr. Tenzin, the local *amji,* or Tibetan herbal doctor, is a short, handsome man of thirty-eight who spent four years at a Tibetan medical school in Lhasa learning to treat patients and to blend the herbal medicines that he prescribes. The pharmaceutical part of his training was crucial, he told me, because a Tibetan healer is not allowed to charge patients for medical care. Rather, he earns a living by selling patients his homemade medications. Dr. Tenzin told me that he has high respect for the Western medicine practiced at the Canadian clinic.

"If someone comes in with a fracture or appendicitis, I send them right to Khunde," Dr. Tenzin said. "That's what Western medicine is good at. On the other hand, the doctors up at Khunde refer patients to me, too. If the problem is something like jaundice or chronic gastritis or allergy, they know that Tibetan medication can help. And why wouldn't we help? We have mantras and herbal medicines that have been curing those diseases for two thousand years. If the problem is mental health, like depression, we doctors sometimes send the patient to the *gompa* [the monastery] for prayer with the lama. That really helps some people."

I couldn't resist the temptation to show Dr. Tenzin my bum right shoulder and its limited movement. Could he help me? He replied that he could make up some custom-blended herbal pills that would probably make a difference. But first he needed to know more about my shoulder problem. As it happened, I had my X-rays right there in my backpack, but I hesitated to show them to an *amji.* Would ancient Tibetan medicine recognize the value of X-rays? "Absolutely!" the doctor said. "When patients bring me their X-rays from the clinic up at Khunde, this is extremely helpful in my treatment." On the other hand, Dr. Tenzin was mystified by other diagnostic practices in Western medicine. "When they do urinalysis up at Khunde, all they do is stick a slip of paper into the sample," he said. "But that can't be enough. I just don't think it is possible to diagnose a medical problem and propose a course of treatment without tasting the urine. Certainly I wouldn't begin a diagnosis of your shoulder until I had tasted your urine. It tells so much about a patient's health status."

After the doctor carried out his Tibetan-style urine sample, he got into the familiar palpation and manipulation of my shoulder, discussing the situation all the while with his wife, a fellow *amji*. Eventually, he told me that a regimen of herbal medication, which he would mix up on the spot, would help significantly to reduce pain and increase movement in my injured joint. And then he gave me a mantra to recite each time I took the daily dose of medicine. I must have raised my eyebrows at that, because the friendly *amji* now turned rather stern. Only a fool, he said, would buy and take the medicine without saying the mantra that was essential to its effectiveness. In the end, I bought the medicine—it cost about $4 for two weeks' dosage. I took the medicine, reciting the mantra each time. All this had no discernible effect on my shoulder, positive or negative. But at least I had the money to pay Dr. Tenzin; I didn't have time to paint his clinic.

THAT EXPERIENCE PREPARED ME somewhat for my interaction with Ayurveda at the Arya Vaidya Chikitsalayam. Accordingly, I raised minimal objections with the *vaidyas* about the astrology, the temple visits, the boring diet, and the vile daily medicines that were required elements of shoulder treatment in India. Over the weeks of traditional Indian medicine and massage, I got into a mellow, new-age frame of mind. Certainly the price was right; my stay at the *chikitsalayam*, including a small suite with its own dedicated massage chamber, all treatment, all medication, and all the *dal bhat* I could eat, was priced at $42.85 per night—about what they charge you for a new toothbrush in an American hospital. The explanation for that rock-bottom fee is partly India's minimal cost of living and partly the Out-of-Pocket Model of health care. Treatment at Ayurvedic clinics like the Arya Vaidya, including the yajnopathic diagnosis, is generally covered by Indian health insurance plans. But there are so few Indians who have insurance coverage that most domestic patients pay out of pocket. Accordingly, the clinic has to hold prices down to bargain-basement levels.

In some ways, the *vaidyas* looked like Western doctors; they wore white coats, with stethoscopes draped around their necks, and walked around the hospital's leafy campus with patients' X-rays under their arms. But their view of medicine was strikingly different from what you'd find back home at Johns Hopkins or Mayo. This became clear in my first hour of treatment, when I was examined by an earnest, thoughtful doctor named Ram Manohar.

He used a stainless-steel protractor to measure the range of movement in my right shoulder. "There is significant restriction of angular rotation," he said, speaking the clipped, precise English of educated Indians. "The situation is dismal." He was right, of course, but I didn't like hearing it from a doctor. I asked a pointed question: "So, do you think you can cure this?" The answer was just as pointed: "Oh, I'm not going to cure anything," Dr. Manohar said.

"This is not how Ayurveda works," the doctor went on. "The doctor is not your healer. Ayurveda is based on the conviction that your body knows how to cure itself. I'm not going to cure you; your body will do that. Ayurveda believes that there is a flow of energy through the body—we call it *prana*—and that keeps your body in balance. The reason you have trouble in your shoulder is that the natural forces—we call them the *doshas*—are out of balance. What our treatment will do is restore the flow of *prana*. Then your *doshas* will rebalance and your shoulder condition will improve. But in Ayurveda, the body, not the doctor, manages the healing process."

The body's natural power to heal itself was the core discovery of the ancient doctors who developed Ayurvedic medicine a couple of millennia ago. As related in the Hindu scriptures, the Vedas, the early sages made a careful study of the human body, in the way mechanics might study a car or a locomotive. They concluded—at a time when average life expectancy in India was probably around four decades— that this natural machine was built to last one hundred years, and would do so if properly maintained. The body of medical practice that grew from this work became known as Ayurveda, a Sanskrit word that means "the study of longevity." (In India, it is generally pronounced "eye-yur-WAY-dah.") The inventors of Ayurveda found hundreds of herbs and other plants with medicinal properties to help the body generate *prana*. To make sure that this healing energy force could flow freely through bodily passages, they developed a form of exercise known as yoga. Americans these days flock to yoga classes for fitness and weight control, but in its homeland the purpose of yoga is to eliminate internal blockages so that the body's natural energy can flow and heal. Another prescribed methodology for unblocking the body is Ayurvedic massage, a powerful tool in which the masseur uses medi-cated oils and his own powerful hands to open and smooth the bodily routes that the *prana* needs to follow.

At the hands of Dr. Manohar and other earnest, committed *vaidyas,* my treatment involved all those elements. Six times each day I was required to imbibe a vile assortment of herbal medicines, most of which tasted like spoiled greens or aging mud. Several times I was told to attend the temple on the hospital grounds to perform *poojah,* or reverence, to the Hindu god of healing, Dhanwanthari. I was given various yogic exercises to perform. I was repeatedly ordered to relax, to forget whatever stresses and worries I might have left back home.

"The basic rule is 'Don't think too much,'" Dr. Manohar told me. Still, I was urged to read one of the key Hindu scriptures, the Bhagavad Gita, which turned out to be the inspiring tale of a ruler who loses his courage on the battlefield until the god Vishnu appears and offers one of history's greatest sermons on the theme of "Never surrender." Thus inspired, I refused to surrender to skepticism or hostility, even as I confronted one of the less desirable aspects of the regimen: the hospital diet. To spare my body from expending its energy on digestion, I was restricted to a bland and unchanging menu of rice topped with lentil sauce. This insipid dish is known in South Asia as *dal bhat,* but I soon adopted the nickname for it used by the other Western inmates of the *chikitsalayam:* "dull butt."

The sweetest part of Indian medicine came three times a day, when I lay down for an oil massage at the hands of my strong, skillful therapists, Vinodh and Balu. Like a chicken being readied for the rotisserie, I was stretched on a long black slab of neem wood and marinated in a warm sesame oil laced with forty-six herbs and medications. (The formula for this oil was first set down about 500 BC in a work called the *Ashtanga Hridayam.* Ayurvedic pharmacists have stuck to that ancient recipe ever since.) Vinodh would chant a prayer to Dhanwanthari and then start in, working meticulously on every oiled limb and every muscle in my body. He massaged every finger and every toe; he cracked every knuckle; he massaged my eyelids and earlobes. He used long, powerful strokes that moved smoothly from my right shoulder to my left heel and vice versa. As those strong hands flowed over me, I could almost feel the blocked channels in my body opening up to release the flow of *prana.* This full-body workout, known as *abhyangam,* was followed by a localized massage, or *pizhichil,* of my bad shoulder, using even warmer oil and even stronger massage. While Balu dripped the medicated oil over my joint, Vinodh's forceful fingers would go to work.

These daily rubdowns left the patient feeling marvelous—but they also left me drenched in oil from hair to soles. The solution to that problem was almost as good as the massage. After the morning sessions, Vinodh would wash me all over with a soupy soap made of ground green beans. This ritual removed all the oil and left me smelling like a fresh legume straight from the garden.

Each afternoon, Vinodh and Balu would return to my massage table for the strangest treatment of all, an ancient procedure called *navaraki-zhi*. One man would immerse fist-sized burlap bags filled with rice in a vat of boiling milk; then the other would use those heated rice bags to smite and knead my back and shoulder. Dr. Manohar told me that ancient scripture recommended *navarakizhi* as a way to revive debilitated muscle tissue. It sounded far-fetched, but so what? It felt great.

In this stress-free, unhurried, low-cal way, I spent a few weeks undergoing Ayurvedic treatment at the *chikitsalayam*. As I got into the Ayurvedic life, I began wearing a dhoti, the Gandhi-style wrapound skirt for men. I reread the Bhagavad Gita several times. I could almost feel my *doshas* floating back into balance. And gradually, I began to realize that all this ancient medicine was working.

ON THE LAST DAY of my stay at the *chikitsalayam,* Dr. Ram Manohar came in, accompanied by two of the younger *vaidyas,* with their white coats and stethoscopes and measuring tapes. It was time to assess the results of my treatment, to see whether ancient Indian medicine had brought about any improvement in the bum shoulder of a skeptical modern-day American. By that point, though, I already knew the answer.

For once, Dr. Manohar was silent. Dr. Hemalata, a youthful *vaidya* so petite she had to tilt her head upward just to look at my shoulder, started asking questions. "How is your pain?" she queried. "As a matter of fact," I said, "I don't have any pain in my shoulder. I began to notice that a few days ago. The pain I normally feel when I wake up is gone.

My shoulder feels fine." This moved Dr. Hemalata to a broad, satisfied smile, so pretty and so infectious that I started smiling, too. Then she took out Dr. Manohar's stainless-steel medical protractor; she told me to raise my right arm as high as I could and measured the angle of rotation in my shoulder. "There is significant increase in range of motion," she said, her smile growing even broader. "Your shoulder is greatly improved." As if that weren't good enough, the *vaidyas* then led me to a scale; under the relentless regimen of massage and the relentless diet of *dal bhat,* I had lost nine pounds in a matter of weeks. But even that stellar achievement paled compared to the obvious improvement in my frozen joint.

To this day, I don't know why it happened: Was it the massage, the medication, the meditation, or Mrs. Rama and her star charts? In any case, the timing was definitely propitious. Ayurveda worked for me. I didn't have a miracle cure; my shoulder was not completely healed. But my pain decreased, my range of motion increased, and I was definitely better—and all without the trouble or cost of a total shoulder arthroplasty. When the front office at the Arya Vaidya Chikitsalayam handed me a detailed accounting—dozens and dozens of pages listing every *navarakizhi,* every *poojah,* and every ancient herbal medication I had experienced—I realized instantly that my U.S. insurance company was never going to pay this bill. But my experience with traditional Indian medicine was so positive that I had no regrets about paying the whole thing, out of pocket.

TEN

Too Big to Change?

THE MODELS WE'VE SEEN IN THE WORLD'S OTHER WEALTHY, industrialized democracies could pave the way for reform of the U.S. health care system. All the countries like us have already made the essential moral decision—every person shall have access to a doctor when needed—and all of them have developed mechanisms to make that guarantee a reality. As we've seen, all the other rich countries provide high-quality, universal care, and yet they spend far less than the United States does. Which means that we need only borrow a few good ideas, from this country or that one, to arrive at reasonably priced universal coverage for the USA. It sounds so simple.

In fact, though, revamping a nation's health care system is never simple. American history is replete with proof of that unhappy truth. From Theodore Roosevelt to Barack Obama, half a dozen U.S. presidents have come to office promising "health care reform" and "universal coverage." President Bill Clinton made health care a central issue of his successful campaign in 1992. Once in office, he announced in his first State of the Union Address that health care reform would be his chief domestic priority. "All of our efforts to strengthen the economy will fail unless we take bold steps to reform our health care system," the newly elected Clinton told Congress, punching the air with his fist for emphasis.

But the ambitious Clinton reform effort flopped; indeed, it never even came to a vote in Congress. There were several explanations for that defeat, ranging from Bill and Hilary Clinton's political mistakes to the hidebound nature of America's political institutions. But the most common theory about the failure of the Clinton reform plan—and of the Roosevelt, Wilson, Truman, and Nixon reform plans before it—involved the nature of health care itself. This line of analysis holds that the business of providing and paying for Americans' medical care is so complex and involves so much money that significant change is politically hopeless. The arguments quickly focus on which interests might win and which might lose under a given plan. In the process, the basic moral question that should drive reform—do we want to give everybody access to health care?—gets swept aside.

That same pattern was repeated when President Barack Obama took up health care reform at the start of his presidency. Facing an entrenched army of well-financed and powerful interests determined to preserve the status quo, Obama declared from the start that he would not seek to replace the existing health care system with a simpler, cheaper model. "We have to build on what we've got already," Obama said. The result was an enormously expensive and complicated piece of legislation—the "Obamacare" bill runs to 2,400 pages of legalese—that retains most of the structure of the U.S. system but will still leave some 23 million people uninsured when it takes full effect in the year 2015.

Given this long history of failed efforts to achieve universal coverage, many Americans have concluded that health care reform is beyond the power of a democratic government. As political analyst Ezra Klein put it, the political history surrounding the issue suggests that "health care is simply too big, too complicated, and too dangerous to touch."[1]

OR IS IT? In every industrialized country, the health care business is a huge and complicated industry, with tens of thousands of participants and untold billions of dollars or euros or yen, etc., at stake. In every wealthy country, there are powerful interests with large investments in the status quo. And yet, as we have seen in this book, other industrialized, free-market democracies have managed to change their health care systems, despite the high stakes and the vested interests. In some nations—France, Germany, the UK, for example—health care "reform" is just about a full-time process, with new rules and adjustments to the system emerging from the parliament every few years or so. Generally, these reforms don't change the basic nature of a national health care system. Britain holds true to the Beveridge Model, even as it tries to introduce some market-style competition among hospitals; Germany still uses the Bismarck Model, but it made a major change in 1993, switching from regional health insurance to national insurance plans that any German can buy.[2]

And yet some industrialized democracies have carried out fundamental reform of their health care systems, despite significant political opposition. In the course of my global quest, I visited two countries that completely revamped their national health care arrangements: Switzerland and Taiwan. Both countries made a national commitment to provide health care to all. Having committed to universal coverage, both democracies were able to bring about the changes necessary to get there.

Neither of these countries looks much like the United States of America, of course. Taiwan is an island nation of 23 million Chinese people with a deep commitment to Confucian traditions. Switzerland has 8 million people steeped in European culture and history, speaking four different official languages. Still, both countries have important parallels to the United States. Both are vigorous democracies marked by fierce competition between political parties that look a lot like our Republicans and Democrats. Both have finance and insurance industries that are rich and politically influential. Both are ferociously capitalist places, and both have jumped aboard the digital revolution to build advanced, high-tech economies. Most important, both Taiwan and Switzerland had fragmented and expensive health care, similar to the American system—until they launched their reform campaigns. In both countries, payment for medical care was dominated by health insurance plans tied to employment; in both, significant numbers of people were left with no coverage at all. Even with large numbers of people uninsured, both countries were pouring considerable amounts of money into health care. In both Taiwan and Switzerland, as in the United States today, a growing chorus of voices began demanding universal coverage, arguing that every sick person should have access to a doctor.

But at that point, the parallels end. The big difference between those two democracies and the United States is that, in Taiwan and Switzerland, the advocates of universal coverage eventually won the day. Both of those nations adopted new health care systems to guarantee that everybody would be covered—and both of them happened to do it in 1994, the same year that the Clinton health care plan was going down in flames. So I went to these countries looking for lessons we might profitably learn about fixing a broken health care system so that it covers everybody.

THE ISLAND THAT the Chinese call Taiwan—written with two characters that mean "great harbor"—was known for centuries as Formosa, or "beautiful island," a name bestowed by early Portuguese explorers.

It is about the same size as Maryland. While much of it is uninhabit-able mountain and forest, the island is still home to 23 million people (Maryland, in contrast, has a population of 6 million). The island was a province of China for centuries, then became a piece of Japan's Asian empire from 1894 until the end of World War II in 1945. The Japanese military ruled harshly but also built roads and hospitals and drained swamps to defeat malaria; as a result, Taiwan is one of the few former Japanese colonies where the schools teach that the colonial era was benign. The island's modern history began in 1949. Having lost the long civil war to Mao Tse-tung and the Communists, the leaders of China's Nationalist Party, the Guomintang, fled the mainland and set up a government on Taiwan. Eventually, 2 million fugitives crossed the Taiwan Strait, and these newcomers from the mainland immediately set up a government of their own, under the dictatorship of the Na-tionalist strongman Generalissimo Chiang Kai-shek.

Chiang's Nationalists brought with them some of the finest works of art from the mainland's greatest museums. They also brought along the interred remains of China's George Washington, Sun Yat-sen, the leader of the revolution that overthrew the last dynasty in 1911. (Today, there is a lavish tomb and memorial to Sun Yat-sen in Taipei, the cap-ital of Taiwan.) Chiang used these cherished pieces of Chinese history to bolster his claim—which he maintained steadfastly until his death, in 1975—that his Nationalist outpost on Taiwan (the Republic of China) was the real government of China and that the Communist regime which happened to rule a billion Chinese on the mainland (the People's Republic of China) was an impostor with no legitimate claim to power. It was a bizarre geopolitical example of the tail trying to wag the dog, but for two decades, Chiang Kai-shek got most of the world to go along. Not until 1971 did the United Nations eject the Taiwanese and recognize the Communists in Beijing as the legiti-mate government of China. Gradually, almost all the other nations of the world—even the USA, Chiang's strongest bulwark—switched their recognition to the mainland as well. Yet the old argument about who really rules the nation of China still resonates on Taiwan; the residents of the island are debating to this day about what their nation should be called. The Nationalists insist on the name Republic of China and still argue that there is one China. The opposition party, the Democratic Progressives, says the island should declare itself a separate nation called Taiwan and petition the UN for membership under that name.

Whatever its proper name, Taiwan/Republic of China emerged in the late twentieth century as one of the "new Asian Tigers." Following the Japanese model of industrialization, it built a technology-based, export-driven economy that saw explosive growth. Almost overnight— well, over a period of fifteen years, which is the equivalent of the blink of an eye in global economics—Taiwan went from being just another poor country to one of the twenty-five richest nations in the world. Like many other newly rich countries, it also became a democracy. Under intense public pressure, the Nationalist Party that Chiang Kai-shek had founded began to allow open political opposition in the 1980s. Gradually, the liberal, green, pro-labor Democratic Progressive Party emerged as a serious challenger to the pro-business, defense-minded Nationalists. With intensive guidance and subsidies from the government, high-tech industry made Taiwan one of the world's leading producers of microchips, computers, and high-definition audio and video gear. By the early 1990s, Taiwan had the money to build divided highways, bullet trains, state-of-the-art engineering schools, and other accoutrements of an advanced nation.

But it still had a poor country's health care system—which is to say, an out-of-pocket system for most of the people. There were insurance plans for government employees, farmers, soldiers, and employees of some big companies, but 60 percent of the population had no coverage at all. They could see a doctor or go to a hospital only if they could scratch up enough money out of pocket to pay the bill. In a political pattern that would be familiar to Americans, the liberal Democrats latched onto universal health care as a central issue. They made two arguments for universal coverage. On a moral level, the Democrats said, a prosperous country like Taiwan had a basic ethical duty to provide access to medical care for all its people. But there was also the matter of national pride: A national health care system would be one more area in which wealthy Taiwan surpassed mainland China. For some years, the political argument over health care followed predictable left-right lines, with the liberal Democrats agitating for universal coverage and the conservative Nationalists backing the status quo. But in Taiwan, the familiar script took an unexpected turn: The conservative party changed its position. At the same time America's conservative Republicans were going to the mat to defeat the Clinton health care plan, Taiwan's conservative Nationalists took the opposite tack. They endorsed universal coverage, stealing the liberals' strongest issue. In 1994, with strong backing from the Nationalist president, Lee Teng-hui, Taiwan's parliament created a National Health Insurance system that guaranteed coverage for every resident of Taiwan. Largely because of this popular initiative, Lee's conservative party held off the Democrats, and he won the presidency again in 1996.

Taiwan's new health care system was the product of several years of study. In the late 1980s, with the Democratic Progressive Party pressing hard on the issue, President Lee set up a commission to consider health care reform. "The first thing we realized," said Chang Hong-jen, a businessman who was involved in the planning, "was that a little island of 23 million people didn't really know how to run a national health care system. Well, there's a Chinese saying: 'To find your way in the fog, follow the tracks of the oxcart ahead of you.' So we decided the intelligent way through the fog was to look at other industrialized countries. The basic plan was to figure out which nations had found a smart path to universal health care coverage, and follow those tracks." In other words, the Taiwanese did precisely what this book is designed to do: search the developed world for effective health care systems and take lessons from the ones that work best.

To lead them on this global exercise in comparative policy analysis, the Taiwanese hired the best possible tour guide: Professor William Hsiao, a health care economist at the Harvard School of Public Health. Born in Beijing in the 1930s, Hsiao (pronounced like the first syllable of "shower") was the son of a Guomintang official and came to the United States to stay when his father worked with the Taiwanese delegation at the United Nations. He grew up in Queens, became an insurance actuary, and worked his way to the very summit of the profession: chief actuary of the Social Security system. Then he went back to school. He was nearly fifty years old when he got his Ph.D., at Harvard, in the economics of health care systems. In the 1980s, the newly minted economist began an intense study of health care financing and delivery around the world. He was in his sixties when his work finally began to gain international recognition. Today, the white-haired septuagenarian travels the world consulting with the governments of nations rich and poor as they try to improve their health care systems. Hsiao can discuss the details of health care financing in Denmark, Dubai, or Djibouti the way a political consultant discusses the latest poll results in DuPage County. He has helped design systems for numerous countries. If you ask Bill Hsiao about some new approach to health care finance, he tends to say, "Yeah, we tried that in Colombia for a while," or "We thought about that for Cyprus, but I decided it wouldn't work." Hsiao's famous textbook, *Getting Health Reform Right,* is required reading among health officials anywhere on earth who are trying to fix a health care system in an era of skyrocketing costs. For a newly rich Asian island nation that needed a health care system built from scratch, Bill Hsiao was just what the doctor ordered.

"Sometime in the late 1980s," Hsiao recalled later, in his lilting, accented English, "the president's office, or the premier's office, or whatever, called me and asked me to lead a task force to give Taiwan a

twenty-first-century health system. I suggested that they study successful systems elsewhere, and they agreed; they knew that old saying, you
know, follow the other guy's oxcart. Where I began was, I commis-
sioned papers from academic leaders in about six advanced nations—
that's Japan, United States, Canada, Germany, Great Britain, and France.
And I asked them each to write a paper: 'What is your country's health
system? What part is successful? Which part is not working well? And
why doesn't it work well?' And then we had a conference in Taipei, over
three days, and all these people debated each other. And I required
cabinet ministers in Taiwan to chair the various sessions, like the minister of finance, the minister of planning, of health. See, when you chair
a meeting, you have to sit through the whole thing and listen. That's
how you educate decision makers."

Then as now, Taiwan's strongest ally and its military defender was
the United States, so the island nation looked hard at health care
mechanisms in the world's richest country. "We have enormous respect
for America," recalls Chang Hong-Jen, the businessman who served on
the planning commission, "and people said, 'Let's do whatever the
Americans do.' But you know, we have a lot of Taiwanese natives who
are practicing medicine in the United States. And they told us that the
U.S. health care system doesn't work for everybody. American health
care is not really a system at all. It's a market. In a market, people with
money can buy what they want and many people are left out. So we
thought, no, we don't want market-driven health care. We want a real
system, something that covers everybody and doesn't depend on how
much money you have."

Considering different recipes from around the world, Hsiao's task
force set out to build a health care system on the Chinese-menu
principle—this part from column A, this part from column B, and so
on. Although Hsiao is a fan of Britain's National Health Service, he
rejected that approach on the grounds that Taiwan had mostly private
hospitals and it had health insurance plans in place already for civil

servants and others. This dictated a model based on private providers and an insurance system to pay the bills. That approach, of course, sounds like the Bismarck Model, as found in Japan and Germany. But Hsiao was not a fan of the way Bismarck countries relied on many different funds to pay the bills. He urged Taiwan to set up a single national insurance system: "When you have a single payer . . . for the doctors and hospitals, then you can identify who's really abusing the system. That also allows you to put a global budget in place. When you have a single payer, you can say, 'I'm only going to spend X percent of my GDP for health insurance,' and you can enforce that."

So Taiwan built a system that uses private doctors and hospitals, with a single, government-run insurance plan to pay them. That's national health insurance—which is to say, the Canadian model. But Hsiao insisted on one major break from the Canadian system: In Taiwan, National Health Insurance is not funded through general taxation; rather, the money people pay to finance the health insurance fund is called a premium. Both employer and employee are required to chip in monthly to pay this "premium." For Hsiao, the nomenclature is important. Yes, there's a mandatory payment for everybody. Yes, it's withheld from pay and goes directly to the government. But this payment is not a tax. "You never want to call it a tax," Hsiao says. "If you call it a national insurance premium, then you're asking people to pay for a product, not to pay a tax to some huge government entity."

Meanwhile, high-tech Taiwan saw the *carte vitale* in France and decided to give all 23 million Taiwanese patients their own electronic card, with medical and billing records embedded on a chip. As in the Bismarck countries, Taiwan made health insurance mandatory for everybody—with government providing interest-free loans to help people who couldn't pay the premium—and guaranteed that anybody, healthy or sick, would be covered. As in France and Japan, the government's newly created Bureau of National Health Insurance was given central power to set the prices for medical services and drugs. And as in France and Japan, this has proven to be a powerful force in keeping prices low. Because the health insurance plan is run by the government and is thus highly responsive to political pressure, Taiwan's plan covers just about every imaginable form of medical treatment, including physical, mental, dental, and optical, as well as organ transplants, acupuncture, Chinese massage, drugs, traditional herbal medicines, and long-term care.

In early 1993, just as the Clinton reform effort was launched in the United States, Hsiao's commission finished its plan and presented its proposal to the Parliament. After extensive debate, the National Health Insurance Law was passed in July of 1994, with support from both the Democrats and the Nationalists. Hsiao and his planners had expected five years of planning and setup time before the system opened for business. But President Lee was determined to have universal health care in place well before the 1996 presidential election, so his Nationalist government could take the credit. Sure enough, Taiwan's National Health Insurance system began offering universal coverage on March 1, 1995.

Almost overnight, some 11 million Taiwanese who had no medical insurance suddenly had access to doctors and hospitals, with the Bureau of National Health Insurance paying most of the bill. This created a flood of new demand for medical services. The market responded with a flood of new supply: Clinics, hospitals, dentists, optometrists, labs, hostels, and acupuncture centers sprang up everywhere. It was not exactly the way a Harvard economist might have planned it, but Bill Hsiao says now that things worked out reasonably well. "We had this sudden explosion of new suppliers," Hsiao told me during an inspection visit to Taiwan a dozen years after his project was launched. "And that has meant lots of competition, lots of access for the people, and low prices." The government insurance allows patients free choice of any hospital, clinic, or doctor, so providers end up competing furiously for customers. Many clinics offer free ambulance service to bring the patient to the examining room. In most Taiwanese cities, medical clinics stay open twelve hours a day, seven days a week. The doctors don't particularly like it, but they have to operate that way. After all, their competitors down the street are open for business. Chang Hong-Jen, the businessman who helped design the system—and later became the CEO of the Bureau of National Health Insurance—told me that "doctors in Taiwan work very, very hard, because they have to use volume to make up for the low fees."

The most striking result of Taiwan's new system is a healthier population with a longer healthy life expectancy and much higher recovery rates from major diseases. This is particularly evident in rural areas, where it was difficult or impossible to see a doctor before the new system took place. In the fishing village of Jinshan, on a rocky shoreline along Taiwan's east coast, the local government built a hospital at the turn of the twenty-first century. It was the first hospital Jinshan ever had, and it was possible only because National Health Insurance could pay the bills. In 2007, when I visited the place with Professor Hsiao, we got a personal, human reminder of the impact of universal health coverage. In the hospital lobby, a woman named Lee Ching-li was checking people's blood pressure while they waited to see the doctor. Mrs. Lee told me that she wasn't a hospital employee; she just came over a few mornings each week as a volunteer. "Why do you volunteer?" I asked her. Mrs. Lee explained: Her mother contracted breast cancer in the 1980s, when Taiwan had no national health care system and Jinshan had no hospital. Her mother died. Some twenty years later, Mrs. Lee also got breast cancer, and feared the worst. By then, though, Jinshan had its new hospital and Taiwan had a health care system that ensured treatment for Lee Ching-li. She recovered completely. She expects to live forty years longer than her mother did, to see her children and grandchildren grow to adulthood. She felt a need to express her gratitude to the doctors, the hospital, and the system that cured her, so now she volunteers three days a week at the hospital.

When Mrs. Lee finished her story, I pointed across the lobby at Professor Hsiao. "Right over there," I said, "is the guy who set up the health care system that treated your cancer." Hesitantly, bashfully, Mrs. Lee walked over to Bill Hsiao. She told him briefly about her treatment. Then she backed away two steps and gave him a minute nod of the head; a tiny, almost imperceptible bow of gratitude. It was quiet, simple, understated—and to me, the perfect way to say: "Thank you for saving my life."

As a system started from scratch, with uniform rules and procedures for every doctor and patient and state-of-the-art paperless record-keeping, Taiwan's new health insurance system is the most efficient in the world. The 1994 law seemed hopelessly optimistic when it set a limit of 3.5 percent for administrative costs; in fact, the system has done much better than that, with paperwork, etc. accounting for only 2 percent of costs most years (and sometimes less). That's about the same administrative cost rate as in the U.S. Medicare system—but one-tenth as high as the administrative burden for America's private health insurers. As a result, even with explosive growth in the consumption of medical services, national health spending in Taiwan remains at about 6 percent of gross domestic product (as opposed to about 17 percent of GDP in the United States). This has kept costs low for patients. The co-pay for a doctor visit runs about $7; the monthly premium for an entire family's health insurance averages $150 or so.

Indeed, the low rate of spending has emerged as the most serious problem facing Taiwanese health care in the second decade of the national system. Many clinics and hospitals are defaulting on bank loans and threatening to declare bankruptcy unless National Health Insurance agrees to pay higher fees. Since 2002, the Bureau of National Health Insurance—that is, the national government—has had to borrow from banks to pay its bills, because the politicians have been afraid to make their constituents pay higher premiums or co-pays. It seems almost certain that Taiwan will have to increase the health care premiums paid by workers and employers, and perhaps chip in money from general tax revenues to keep the medical providers afloat. In the end, Taiwan may have to pay as much as 8 percent of its GDP for its universal health care system.[3] But even if it gets to that point, Taiwan will be at less than half the U.S. rate of health care spending—while providing coverage for everybody.

The Taiwanese-American economist Tsung-Mei Cheng was one of the experts who helped design Taiwan's health care system. A decade after the National Health Insurance program was established, Cheng prepared a detailed assessment of how it was working—quite well, she said, except for the underfunding—and why Taiwan was able to achieve such a major change.

The plan succeeded, she said, "because of a confluence of several conditions." The primary force for change was the nation's strong feeling on the moral question, Cheng explained. "First, there was a strong public demand for universal health insurance. Second, an entrenched political party with a parliamentary majority found itself challenged by a rising opposition party that had openly embraced universal health insurance. Third, sustained economic growth . . . made financing a major new program feasible. . . . The lesson for policymakers elsewhere is that such windows of opportunity come along only every so often."[4]

IT'S ONE THING, of course, for a newly prosperous nation like Taiwan, with minimal medical infrastructure, to create a wholly new health care system. But the problems take on a whole new dimension when it comes to revamping the established health care system in a thriving, capitalist democracy that has an influential network of health insurance companies, hospitals, and drug companies already in place. In fact, though, a major reform was accomplished—despite the political and economic resistance of a powerful medical industry—in Switzerland. And the "window of opportunity" came along in 1994, the same year that reform was approved in Taiwan and rejected in the USA.

The Swiss Federation is a federal union of twenty-six cantons, or states. They sit in scenic splendor amid high mountain valleys in the heart of Europe, surrounded by Germany, France, Austria, and Italy. While the countries around them have engaged in repeated warfare, the Swiss have remained steadfastly neutral for centuries. That stance has been honored by all the neighbors, because it is useful for the larger, more powerful countries to have a nonaligned entity in their midst. Being neutral means not having enemies, but it also means not having strong allies. As a result, the neutral Swiss are always on the lookout for danger; they spend a good chunk of their federal budget maintaining an army (with mandatory service for all males), and the rate of gun ownership is higher than in the United States. Over the centuries, this Alpine crossroads developed an extensive finance industry— banking, investment, insurance—serving as a safe repository for both commercial profits and criminal plunder from all over Europe. These businesses, combined with a national commitment to education, a penchant for precision manufacturing, and a setting that is ideal for tourism, have made Switzerland one of the richest countries on earth. For decades it has enjoyed per-capita income higher than America's—in 2009, about $41,700 per person.[5]

The Swiss population reflects a range of national and cultural backgrounds. Its 8 million people speak four official languages: German, French, Italian, and Romansch, a Latin derivative. For this reason, a key element of the Swiss national experience is the maintenance of unity, of the sense of belonging, among this diverse population. In the same way that Americans love to invoke concepts like freedom and independence, the Swiss constantly talk about solidarity—or *Solidarität, solidarité,* or *solidarietà.* In Swiss parlance, the word is freighted with many meanings, including "community" and "equal treatment" and "despite our differences, we're all in this together." The president of the Swiss Federation, Pascal Couchepin, explained this idea to me: "In a country of different languages and cultures, we must preserve solidarity. That is why we require that children in our German-speaking cantons learn French and Italian in school; we have similar language requirements in the other regions. We must all talk to each other. And we have this strange government structure—a Federal Council with members from all the parties. We rotate the presidency and the cabinet posts among the parties. This is done to preserve solidarity within our society. Everybody gets an equal chance."

Another definition of "solidarity" in the Swiss context is the principle that all the people of Switzerland should have equal access to basic rights: Everybody gets to vote, everybody gets a jury trial, everybody gets an old-age pension, everybody pays the same price for a ticket on the national railroads. And everybody has access to medical care. In Switzerland, the "right to medical care" is not a political argument advanced by left-wing parties but, rather, a basic truth of modern life. President Couchepin, a corporate executive who became a leading figure in the Christian-Democratic Party—the European version of America's Republicans—set this forth for me, in his excellent but accented English, in dramatic terms. "A society cannot have complete equality," M. Couchepin said. "It is not possible. You can earn more money than your neighbor; that is not society's business. But a good railway system, a good school system, a good health system—the basic needs of the people—must be handled with a high degree of equality. To have a great sense of solidarity among the people, all must have an equal right—and particularly, a right to medical care. Because it is a profound need for people to be sure, if they are struck by the stroke of destiny, they can have a good health system. Our society must meet that need."

In health care, though, the basic solidarity, the equality, of Swiss society became badly strained near the end of the twentieth century. The Swiss health insurance business was coming to resemble the American system. Traditionally, Switzerland had had a network of "mutual," or nonprofit, health insurance plans; workers bought insurance through their employer. But Switzerland is home to some of the world's largest insurance firms. In the 1980s, these private insurance giants learned a profitable lesson from American insurers. U.S. companies like Aetna and UnitedHealth had been buying up nonprofit health insurers like Blue Cross and Blue Shield and converting them into profit-making operations. As it turned out, for-profit health insurance produced fabulous bottom-line results, especially when the insurers were picky about the people they covered and diligent about denying claims. The big Swiss insurance firms were impressed; they started buying the old mutual health plans in Switzerland and converting them into profit-making businesses. By the early 1990s, Switzerland's health care system was the closest in the world to the American model. Costs were high—Switzerland ranked second only to the United States in per-capita spending on health care—and more and more Swiss citizens were being left without insurance. Just as in America, the insurance companies refused to cover anybody with a preexisting condition, on the logical theory that covering sick people would cost more and eat into profits. Even those who had coverage found their claims being denied, because the insurers decided, logically, that every claim they paid would eat into profits.

It was a fine example of unfettered capitalism at work. But in Switzerland, there was a problem. Even more than it cherishes capitalism and profit, Switzerland cherishes its solidarity. And this change in the health insurance market began to undermine solidarity. Some Swiss people could afford to see a doctor when they were ill; others could not. Some people were covered for large medical bills; others faced bankruptcy. By 1993, nearly four hundred thousand Swiss citizens had no health insurance coverage—about 5 percent of the population.[6] By U.S. standards, of course, that would be barely a blip; in 2009, some 16 percent of Americans were living without health insurance. For the Swiss, though, leaving 5 percent of their fellow citizens outside the health care system was an unacceptable violation of the core national values: solidarity, community, equality.

A special task force was set up to study this national problem. The commission examined the transformation of health insurance in Switzerland, but also took a long look at the systems in other European nations. The Beveridge Model was rejected fairly quickly, on the grounds that capitalist Switzerland was not about to turn such a large part of its economy over to a British-style National Health Service. But the Bismarck systems in neighboring France and Germany— relying on private but nonprofit health insurance plans—was closer to Swiss ideals. With strong support from the liberal parties, the commission in 1993 proposed a bold new approach to health insurance, based largely on the Bismarck Model. The new law—the Swiss Federal Law on Compulsory Health Care, or Loi Fédérale sur L'Assurance-Maladie—was dubbed LAMal. This is a French pun—*mal* is French for "illness," but the acronym stands for "health insurance law," from the law's French name. Under this plan, health insurance was separated from employment, and every family went out in the market to buy coverage. Insurance companies were required to offer a basic package of benefits to all applicants, and insurers could not make a profit on basic health coverage (any profits or surplus earnings must be used to reduce premiums for the next year). To soften the impact on the insurance industry, the new law required that everyone buy health insurance; anyone who didn't sign up was automatically assigned to one of the companies, and the premium was deducted from the paycheck. That ensured the insurance companies a large enough pool of customers to keep them solvent. Further, insurers were allowed to make a profit on supplemental coverage—that is, they could sell additional insurance to pay for cosmetic surgery, private rooms in the hospital, and so on. Under this plan, everybody could afford medical care and nobody would go bankrupt paying doctor bills.

It's a basic rule of Swiss democracy that any major policy change must be approved by the people. And so a national referendum was scheduled on LAMal in 1994, just as the Clinton health care plan was sputtering to its death back in America. As in the United States, the reform proposal sparked heated debate, with the for-profit insurance industry, the drug industry, and most of the rest of the business community fiercely opposed. As in the United States, the opposition warned that the reform would make things worse for the majority of people who already had insurance. On the pro-LAMal side, unions, farmers, and liberal parties countered with the argument that universal health care should be an essential element of Swiss solidarity. Pascal Couchepin's Christian-Democratic Party, normally the voice of the business community, took a neutral stance, reluctant to put itself on the wrong side of a basic principle of Swiss culture. In the end, solidarity prevailed, as it generally does in Switzerland. LAMal was passed with a bare majority of the vote, and the new system went into effect on January 1, 1996.

When I visited Switzerland a dozen years later, universal health care coverage was so firmly entrenched as an element of Swiss life that nobody seemed to oppose it anymore. Even M. Couchepin, the conservative businessman who became president, agreed. "Nobody would want to go back to the system before, when some people were locked out of the insurance," he told me. "We have a system now that means everybody, rich or poor, can have the best health care we can provide. It is accepted; it is working. We are happy that we made the changes in 1994."

Switzerland is still a big spender on medicine. It spends about 11 percent of GDP on health care—that's the second-highest spending rate in the world, and roughly the same share as before LAMal was established. But today, everyone in Switzerland is covered by the insurance system; nobody is turned down for coverage, and no claim can be denied if it is signed by a doctor or a hospital. The absence of profit has not meant an absence of competition among insurance companies; on average, Swiss workers have about seventy different plans to choose from. The insurers can't compete on the basic package of benefits, which is determined by the government. They do battle one another on price, on extra benefits, and on user-friendliness. One of the major insurers, Groupe Mutuel, promises to pay every claim within five days; if it misses that deadline, the next month's premium is free. Most firms have used the nonprofit basic health coverage as a sort of loss leader, to draw customers to profitable lines of business, like supplemental health coverage, life insurance, or fire insurance. "We opposed the reform," Pierre-Marcel Revaz, the president of Groupe Mutuel, told me. "But in fact, our insurance industry has thrived with it. Of course, we are Swiss. So we are pleased that everyone in Switzerland now has access to the same package of care." The insurance industry reports higher profits overall than before LAMal was passed.

And yet the impulse for "health care reform" is still alive in Switzerland, driven largely by unions and by the liberal political parties. This reflects the fact that health insurance, while universal, is also expensive; premiums average about $750 per month for family coverage. Many Swiss blame the insurance industry for that. There has been agitation for a single, government-run health insurance plan, like the one Taiwan established. So far, the Swiss have resisted; a referendum in 2007 to establish a government-run single-payer plan was soundly defeated. "Basically, we prefer a private-sector approach to these matters," President Couchepin told me. "We are satisfied with our LAMal, because it relies on private companies but guarantees that all our people will be treated equally when it comes to medical care."

CAN AMERICANS LEARN ANYTHING from the experience of an emerging Asian island nation and an ancient European confederation? The key lesson from both countries is that health care systems can be changed, even in the face of powerful commercial and political interests. And it's easier for nations to make the change if they follow someone else's oxcart—if they study health care systems in other countries to help design a new system for their own people. On the political front, Taiwan and Switzerland followed the same route toward reform: Liberal political parties stepped up the pressure for change to such a level that the conservative parties were unwilling to resist.

Most important, both the Asian nation steeped in Confucian teachings and the European nation built on Judeo-Christian principles came to the same conclusion on the central moral question posed by a health care system. Both countries decided that society has an ethical obligation—as a matter of justice, of fairness, of solidarity—to assure everybody access to medical care when it's needed. The advocates of reform in both countries clarified and emphasized that moral issue much more than the nuts and bolts of the proposed reform plans. As a result, the national debate was waged largely around ideals like "equal treatment for everybody," "we're all in this together," and "fundamental rights" rather than on the commercial implications for the health care industry.

The contrast with the U.S. approach to health care reform is instructive.

President Clinton emphasized economics in selling his plan to the public. "Over the long run," he argued in his first State of the Union address, "reforming health care is essential to reducing the deficit and expanding investment." Clinton named the smartest and most driven member of his White House team, First Lady Hillary Rodham Clinton, to head the Task Force on National Health Care Reform, and she, too, emphasized the economic impact of change. But the economics of change in a $2 trillion industry were hardly attractive to those whose interests were tied to the status quo. The health insurance industry committed tens of millions of dollars to the famously effective "Harry and Louise" TV ads. The hospital industry, the drug industry, and many physicians' groups joined the insurers in opposition. Their campaign was so effective that the Clinton health care plan never even came to a vote in either house of Congress.

Fifteen years later, President Obama initially tried to sell health care reform with the same economic arguments—and ran into largely the same opposition from those who were doing well under the existing health care system. Obama's team struggled mightily to counter people's fear of change. "Under the plan, if you like your current health insurance, nothing changes," the president said over and over. But this argument didn't work. For one thing, most people didn't believe it. Beyond that, the appeal to those who already had health insurance focused on self-interest, and not on the moral obligation to provide health care for others. During his first year in office, Obama rarely if ever invoked the interest of the tens of millions of Americans without health insurance.

Early in 2010, when most pundits had written off health care reform as a lost cause, Obama came back to the issue and convinced his fellow Democrats to make one more effort to pass a bill. During February and March, in the weeks leading up to the ultimate House and Senate votes, the president completely rewrote his speech on health care. Now he talked mainly about the uninsured. "I'm here because of the countless others who have been forced to face the most terrifying challenges in their lives with the added burden of medical bills they can't pay," Obama told a big crowd in Strongsville, Ohio. "That is not the America I believe in and that's not the America that you believe in." During the last hours of debate before the final votes in Congress, Republicans once again talked about "socialism" and "government takeover"; Democrats invoked the moral argument as their chief reason for supporting reform. And the moral issue that drove major change in Taiwan and Switzerland also proved decisive in the United States.

As discussed in Appendix II of this book, Obama's reform bill, the Patient Protection and Affordable Care Act of 2010, will significantly expand health care coverage in the United States. But the 2010 reform did not get us to universal coverage. However, the experience of all the other rich democracies, including Taiwan and Switzerland, should give us confidence that we can in fact reach that goal.

Of course, there are practical arguments as well for universal health care coverage. Universal coverage saves lives, saves money, reduces the rate of abortion. And it promotes preventive medicine. If the health care system covers everybody, then the system has a powerful incentive to keep people healthy. An apple a day keeps the doctor away, and that means universal health care systems have an interest in providing the apples—as we'll see in the next chapter.

ELEVEN

An Apple a Day

WHEN WE THINK ABOUT MEDICAL CARE, WE TEND TO focus on the fate of an individual patient rather than the health of a whole nation. For an individual who is sick, the quality of hands-on medical care—doctors, nurses, X-rays, hospitals, medicine—is a vital concern. The difference between good treatment and bad can literally be a life-or-death issue. This basic truth is dramatized every week on the TV shows about flamboyant doctors who cure lethal diseases with daring surgical interventions (and then duck into the linen closet for a quick tryst with the nurse). But life-saving medical treatment takes place in real life, too, every day. We've all heard of patients pulled back from the brink of death, of severed limbs re-attached by a skillful surgeon, of damaged hearts and livers and shoulders and knees repaired so completely that the patient can leave the hospital and live as if she had never been ill.

And yet, for society as a whole, the medical care provided to individual patients is just one of the factors that determine overall levels of health—and it is not necessarily the most important. Efforts to keep people healthy in the first place generally contribute more to the health of an entire population than the life-saving work of doctors treating individuals one by one. We've always known this as a matter of common sense:"An ounce of prevention is worth a pound of cure." But modern epidemiological studies make it clear that preventive medicine—the discipline sometimes called public health—trumps individual treatment as a means for keeping large numbers of people healthy, wealthy, and wise.

Still, preventive medicine is not easy, and not always popular. Public health campaigns—Eat more fiber! Put down that cigarette!—can very quickly begin to sound like nagging. A public health officer probing how much I'm drinking or how often I exercise impinges on my privacy. At a time when national health care budgets are stretched to the last penny just caring for the sick, it can be hard to find additional money for preventive treatment of those who are healthy.

This means that any health system needs a strong incentive—an economic incentive—to invest in preventive health care. Of course, governments invest in preventive care out of basic altruism; it is government's job, after all, to protect people. But it helps considerably if there is an economic movitation—an incentive structure that encourages the system to invest in prevention. Public health costs money—billions of dollars per year in the major economies—and the return on that spending may not be seen for years or decades. To get serious preventive care, therefore, you need an incentive structure that encourages long-term investment. This is where the national health system comes in.

In a nation with a unified health system that covers everybody—which is to say, all the industrialized democracies of the world except the USA—it clearly benefits both the population and the system to invest in public health. But in a fragmented, multifaceted-system nation like the United States, the economic incentives for preventive care are dissipated. With numerous systems and payers, the temptation is to shift the expense of preventive care to somebody else. America's private, for-profit health insurers—corporations that have to worry about quarterly and annual returns—find it difficult to justify spending money on preventive care that won't save money for years to come. Indeed, an insurance company may see no savings at all from preventive testing or procedures, because the health problem to be avoided may not develop until the patient is over sixty-five and thus covered by Medicare. In a system where health insurance comes with the job and ends when the job ends, the insurer can expect many customers to terminate coverage in a few years. Insurance experts say the average customer stays with the same plan for less than six years,[1] so an insurance executive with his eye on the bottom line has little financial incentive to pay for long-term prevention. American health insurance plans sometimes do cover mammograms and PSA tests and similar preventive measures, but they do it primarily for marketing purposes, to make their plans more attractive to corporate customers.

On occasion, the incentives built into the U.S. health care system are downright perverse. Because awareness of a preexisting condition can lead to higher insurance premiums—or outright denial of coverage—some Americans deliberately avoid physical exams or other medical tests for fear of losing their health insurance. This means they avoid the preventive care that might help control the condition; eventually, they'll have to go to a doctor for treatment, running up vastly higher costs for the system. Beyond that, health insurers are sometimes more likely to pay for treating disease than for preventing it. "Insurers will often refuse to pay $150 for a diabetic to see a podiatrist, who can help prevent foot ailments," the *New York Times* noted. "Nearly all of them, though, cover amputations, which typically cost more than $30,000. Patients have trouble securing [insurance] reimbursement for a $75 visit to the nutritionist who counsels them on controlling their diabetes. Insurers do not balk, however, at paying $315 for a single session of dialysis, which treats one of the disease's serious complications."[2]

In contrast, all the other rich countries I visited on my global odyssey have a powerful economic interest in keeping people well. The reason was set forth vividly by a Scottish politician named John Reid, who served as Britain's health minister—in essence, the chief of the National Health Service—under Tony Blair. John told me exactly why his NHS saw economic value in preventive medicine: "Almost every person in this country is my patient for life. From the minute the line turns blue on your mother's pregnancy test until the minute you die, maybe ninety-nine years later, you are my patient. If you become ill, it is the job of the NHS to treat you, without regard to cost. So of course I want to prevent you from becoming ill."

EVEN WITH THAT SORT of incentive structure, public health generally doesn't receive the kind of attention that is paid to hands-on medicine. Dramatic surgical advances and biological breakthroughs that lead to new wonder drugs tend to draw the headlines and win the science prizes. In fact, though, the long slog of extended observation and population studies carried out by unsung public health experts generally adds more to the span of our lives. Public health officials frequently point to two key discoveries, both announced in 1953, that crystallize the difference:

- In February, at the Cavendish Laboratory of Cambridge University, the American biologist James Watson and the British physicist Francis Crick figured out the double-helix structure of deoxyribonucleic acid, DNA. That discovery demonstrated how DNA carries and passes on each human being's hereditary information. "We have found the secret of life," Crick said. This wildly celebrated biological advance led to the Nobel Prize, a No. 1 best seller (Watson's memoir, *The Double Helix*), and the science of genomics, which may someday cure chronic diseases and spawn a new world of individualized drugs designed to save people who have a genetic disposition for a lethal illness.

• In November, a German-born American doctor named Ernst L. Wynder read a short paper at the annual meeting of the American Cancer Society. Working with his mentor, Dr. Evarts Graham (a heavy smoker who later died of lung cancer), at Washington University in St. Louis, Wynder had noticed an amazing statistical correlation between habitual smoking and lung cancer. At a time when cigarettes were still promoted on health grounds ("Three out of four doctors recommend Lucky Strike!"), this was a shocking and fiercely controversial finding. The tobacco companies said it was a statistical quirk. There was no scientific evidence, they noted, that linked their products with any disease. To test the accuracy of the statistical data, Wynder devised an ingenious experiment. He built a machine that could inhale cigarettes and capture the tar from condensed tobacco smoke. He then painted this tar on the skin of laboratory rats. The rats died of cancer at unprecedented rates. In that 1953 paper, "The Place of Tobacco in Lung-Cancer Etiology,"[3] Wynder reported his findings. Beyond conjecture, the laboratory evidence confirmed the connection between smoking and cancer. This discovery won no Nobel Prize and produced no best sellers, but it did lead to the surgeon general's warning on every pack of cigarettes and sparked a global public health campaign that has dissuaded hundreds of millions of people from smoking.

A half century later, the famous biological breakthrough of Watson and Crick has deeply enhanced our knowledge of heredity. It holds great promise for health benefits—sometime in the future. Meanwhile, the obscure, largely forgotten public health breakthrough of Ernst L. Wynder has already spared millions of people who would have contracted lung cancer and died prematurely. It has saved huge sums of money that would have been spent to treat all those cancer cases. This is the power of preventive medicine; it saves lives by the million, and dollars, yen, euros, etc., by the billion.

Those uncelebrated doctors who devote their talents to keeping large populations well sometimes look with envy at the stature and income of prizewinning medical researchers and highly paid physicians practicing one-on-one medical treatment. "The prestige of any given specialty within the house of medicine is inversely proportional to the size of the object it addresses," wrote Dr. Ichiro Kawachi, of the Harvard School of Public Health. "Hence if your chosen field of specialty happens to deal with microscopic objects like chromosomes and genes, you can be assured of high prestige as well as unlimited access to funding. If, on the other hand, your chosen field happens to deal with the opposite end of the spectrum from genes—that is, the health of entire populations—then you had better resign yourself to a life of chronic under-funding, low prestige, and being ignored by the rest of the world."[4]

THERE ARE TWO BASIC APPROACHES to the job of keeping people healthy: the Public Health Model and the Medical Model. The first deals with populations as a whole and can involve changing a nation's social and cultural norms on a massive scale. The second approach deals with people on an individual basis, seeking to head off diseases or detect them before they become serious.

THE PUBLIC HEALTH MODEL

In its most ambitious form, the public health approach to preventive medicine deals with fundamental socioeconomic facts of life. For example, poverty is associated with higher rates of illness in every society; poor people get sick more often and die at a younger age than those with an average or high income. In the United States, people with a yearly income below $10,000 are three to six times as likely to die before the age of sixty-four as those with an income over $25,000.[5] Americans living at or near the poverty line are more likely to get cancer than their richer neighbors, and more likely to die within five years of contracting the disease. The variation in health due to wealth or the lack of it is less pronounced in nations that give everybody cheap or free access to medical care; but even in Britain, a country that has eliminated doctor bills, poor people tend to be sicker than the rest of the population.

As if eliminating poverty weren't enough of a challenge for a public health officer, other basic elements of modern life also undermine a nation's overall wellness. Air and water pollution contribute to numerous chronic diseases. But pollution is a by-product of industrial societies. People who travel to work or to the store by foot or bicycle tend to be thinner and healthier than the majority who commute by car or train. But tens of millions of people can't get to work or to the mall without a car, because they live in suburbs that were designed around the automobile, with housing placed miles away from any shop or office. The stress of overwork is a proven contributor to ill health; those European countries that require employers to offer four, five, or six weeks of paid vacation each year tend to have lower rates of physical and mental disease than the workaholic USA. Many experts argue that violent crime, particularly gun crime, is a major public health problem for young people in the United States. "A strong and statistically significant association exists between gun availability and death rates" among people under twenty-four, one study concludes.[6] (As we saw in chapter 6, experts who have studied public health in Japan, the nation with the world's longest healthy life expectancy, agree that the extremely low crime rate there is a contributor to its enviable health statistics.) It is well-known that high-salt, high-sugar, high-fat foods promote diabetes, coronary heart disease, various cancers, and other chronic health problems. For the United States—home of the Whopper, the stuffed-crust pizza, the glazed doughnut, and the hot fudge sundae—the ubiquitous fast-food menu is a public health menace.

To eliminate all these threats to the health of the U.S. population, the underfunded, low-prestige public health office in the basement of your local city hall would have to bring about fundamental changes in industry, transit, urban design, work habits, diet, distribution of wealth, and the Second Amendment. In short, the job of preventive medicine can be huge.

But the Public Health Model can also produce huge benefits, as history has proven. When the bubonic plague, the "Black Death," reached Italy in the fourteenth century, officials in Genoa imposed a rule that all arriving ships had to anchor outside the port for a *quarantina*—that is, a period of forty days.[7] This proved so successful in preventing the spread of the disease that isolation, or "quarantine," became a standard tool for containing the plague—a public health intervention that saved millions from painful death in other cities that adopted the practice. In the nineteenth century, public health measures drastically reduced the spread of viruses and bacteria that caused infectious disease. We tend to think that twentieth-century medicine, like vaccinations and antibiotics, conquered such diseases as measles, scarlet fever, whooping cough, and tuberculosis; in fact, there was a sharp decrease in death rates from these ancient killers decades before the wonder drugs came along. Most of the credit goes to public health advances in water purification, sewage disposal, and pasteurization of milk.

For the mass prevention of disease, mass education is a key weapon. That is why health ministries around the world put up huge posters and place ads on TV that ask—or, perhaps, nag—people to eat properly, to get enough exercise, to wash their hands before eating and brush their teeth after. When our children went to public school in Japan, they were taught, along with language and geography and arithmetic, that they must brush their teeth after every meal. This was a law, like gravity. That part of the curriculum was an ambitious effort by the Ministry of Health to deal with the fact that the Japanese, well into the second half of the twentieth century, had a disproportionate number of dental problems. Clearly, the lessons took. Today, virtually every Japanese worker keeps a toothbrush in her desk drawer or in the pocket of his uniform; companies like Sony and Coca-Cola pass out free toothbrushes on the street, for advertising; and in any office building the bathrooms are crowded after every lunch hour with people vigorously brushing. The decline in tooth and gum diseases has been dramatic. In many African countries, the battle against HIV-AIDS relies largely on public education programs. Uganda's famous "ABC" campaign—involving constant repetition of the mantra "**A**bstain, **B**e faithful, use **C**ondoms"—is given much of the credit for the sharp decline in AIDS deaths there in the 1990s.

Ernst L. Wynder's warning that smoking causes fatal disease has prompted health ministries all over the world to mount educational campaigns about the risk of tobacco. More than a hundred nations today require a health warning on every pack of cigarettes and in every tobacco advertisement (in Britain, the warning must be printed in a larger font than any other text in the ad). Although the gist of these messages is similar everywhere, the specific language on cigarette packs tends to reflect each nation's culture and traditions.

In the United States, the surgeon general's warning first appeared in 1966. After extended negotiations with the tobacco industry, the wording was tentative: "Caution: Cigarette Smoking May Be Hazardous to Your Health." Over the years, the warning has grown more specific. Cigarettes sold in America today carry one of several health alerts on the side of the pack, such as "SURGEON GENERAL'S WARNING: Smoking Causes Lung Cancer, Heart Disease, Emphysema, And May Complicate Pregnancy." That's much stronger than the original formula, but still a powder puff compared to what other nations require.

The Brits are blunt about it; their warning is a large white square on both the front and the back of the pack with two words in bold black letters: "Smoking kills." That threat has now become a standard for members of the European Union, so that French smokers are reminded, on the front of the pack, that "Fumer tue"; in Italy, it's "Il fumo uccide"; in Portugal, "Fumar mata"; in Sweden, "Rökning dödar." Germany's warnings are also harsh, such as "Rauchen ist tödlich" ("Smoking is deadly"). In Austria, the label can use a potential form, "Rauchen kann tödlich sein" ("Smoking can be deadly"), which makes the smoker's death seem a little less certain. (This must appeal to a trucker who smokes while behind the wheel making a delivery from, say, Munich, Germany, down to Salzburg, Austria: As long as he is in Germany, he's a dead man driving, but if he makes it across the River Salz into Austria, he has a fighting chance to live.) The Canadians fill cigarette packs with alarming statistics: "85% of lung cancers are caused by smoking. 80% of lung cancer victims die within three years," one required warning label says, in both English and French. Canada also requires a drawing of a lung pocked with cancerous tumors. In Venezuela, the homeland of macho, the warning hits home for the young men who do most of the smoking: "Fumar causa impotencia en los hombres," which is to say "Smoking makes men impotent." In polite Japan, where blunt language like that is generally considered a serious social error, the tobacco warning (on the side of the pack) reflects the nation's ingrained habit of saying everything softly: "Honorable customer, because there is a concern about risk to your honorable health, let's be careful about smoking too much," the label says. With the Japanese concern for social harmony, the warning goes on to suggest, "Let's remember good manners when smoking."[8]

When educational measures are considered inadequate, colleges, companies, and governments move to rules, regulations, and laws to enforce preventive measures. State laws requiring that motorcycle riders wear helmets or that drivers buckle up reflect a sense that education alone is not enough to prevent many preventable injuries. Baby seats in rental cars, hard hats at construction sites, safety locks on shotgun triggers, child-proof pill bottles, a mandatory closing time for bars—these are all examples of public health and safety precautions forced upon people whether they want to be careful or not. The United States has lots of these regulations, but other countries go much further along the road toward Big Brotherism. Singapore installs a warning beeper in your car that goes off in maddening fashion whenever you exceed 55 miles per hour. Japanese schools issue required guidelines for each child's desk, chair, and lamp at home, so that homework won't cause back or vision problems; at the start of the school year, teachers come around to students' homes to make sure these requirements are met. In many French schools, students identified as overweight are required to report to the nurse's office at regular intervals to be weighed. In Taiwan, people considered obese receive a New Year's card from the health ministry, telling them how much weight they are expected to lose in the coming year.

Underlying all these efforts at education, persuasion, and regulation is a basic public health principle: Much of our involvement with medical treatment, whether it's for an illness or an accident, is actually preventable. If you had stopped smoking years ago—or never started in the first place—you probably wouldn't need heroic and expensive treatment today for lung cancer or emphysema. If you had resisted all those French fries and doughnuts, you wouldn't be diabetic. If you had controlled your speed on the ski slope, you wouldn't have broken that leg. If you'd had your toddler properly strapped into a child seat, you wouldn't have to rush him to the emergency room after a minor fender bender. In short, the Public Health Model is built around an impolite message: If you're sick, it may be your own fault. If you or your child is injured, you may have brought it on yourself. Put another way, a key role of any public health regime is to enhance each individual's commitment to personal responsibility.

But if your disease is your fault, who should pay for your medical treatment? In countries where there is a single pool of public money to pay for medical care—Britain's National Health Service, for example, or America's Medicare system for the elderly—the cost of everybody's health care is shared by everybody else. That means some other guy's irresponsible acts can cost me money. A person who smokes or eats too much ice cream or rides a motorcycle without a helmet may be endangering his own body, but he also endangers my wallet. He could be imposing high costs on the health care system, a system funded by my premiums or my tax payments. Does this, in turn, give me the right to nag my neighbor into eating better, drinking less, driving safer? This is the Nanny State problem. It looms large in Britain, where the NHS is like the village green—a common asset that everyone can use and everyone pays for.

In recent years, the British have been engaged in a weighty national debate about obesity, with statistics showing more and more Britons getting fat. (Not surprisingly, the London tabloids have found a way to blame this on America: It's all those snack foods the bloody Yanks are exporting to Britain.) Naturally, the political parties have taken up the argument with gusto. The Conservatives insist that watching one's waistline and keeping in shape is a matter of personal responsibility, and it is the fault of the Labour Party that so many Brits have let personal responsibility go by the wayside. Labour politicians respond that the real issue is corporate greed, with executives in the food, restaurant, and beer industries foisting their fatty products upon unwary consumers through relentless advertising campaigns. Whoever is to blame, the Brits recognize that more obese British people means more expense for the tax-supported NHS.

THE MEDICAL MODEL

This approach to preventive medicine uses the familiar one-on-one system of medical care, with a nurse or doctor treating an individual patient. In preventive care, though, the goal is not to cure a person's disease but to take steps in advance to keep the individual from contracting the disease in the first place. In some cases, these individual interventions are the only effective form of prevention. While many contagious diseases were largely contained by public health measures like sanitation and sewage systems, ailments like smallpox, polio, and tetanus cannot be stopped that way; they require immunization of individual patients. When a doctor notes her patient's weight, cholesterol level, and blood pressure and then unleashes a stern lecture about the need for less fat, more fiber, less alcohol, and more exercise, this is preventive medicine on a personal level. The Medical Model also involves diagnostic testing—the Pap smear to detect cervical cancer, the mammogram for breast cancer, the PSA blood test for prostate cancer, the dreaded colonoscopy for colon cancer—to spot potential diseases while they are still treatable.

For the patient, diagnostic testing is surely a plus. If you have cancer, it's obviously best to get tested and find out early. Even if the test comes back negative, you've gained some peace of mind. For a health system, though, the cost-benefit ratio of extensive testing and preventive procedures is not so clear. Different systems come to different conclusions about which tests to pay for. As we saw in chapter 6, my local government in Japan gave me a comprehensive physical exam every year, with the full range of blood tests, an EKG, and a barium enema. This was provided for free, to me and to every resident of Japan, because the health ministry there decided the cost of the test would pay off in reduced costs for treatment down the road. But when we moved to Britain, the NHS never agreed to provide an annual physical, or even the prostate cancer test that should be standard for a man my age. The Brits have decided that these diagnostic interventions don't provide enough preventive benefit to justify their cost. Britain's National Institute for Health and Clinical Excellence (that is, NICE, the outfit we met in chapter 7) has concluded that giving standard tests for blood pressure, urine, and so on when a patient comes into the doctor's office is as effective as a full-scale physical examination, and cheaper than herding everybody in for a physical every year.

THE DISAGREEMENT ABOUT which tests and procedures are cost-effective gets to an important point about preventive medicine: It can deter disease, it can save lives, it can save money for a health care system—but not always. "Preventing illness can in some cases save money, but in other cases it can add to health costs," noted a 2008 survey of the literature in the *New England Journal of Medicine*.[9] "For example, drugs used to treat high cholesterol yield much greater value for the money if the targeted population is at high risk for coronary heart disease." But if you give anti-cholesterol drugs to people who aren't high-risk candidates, the cost of "prevention" turns out to be more than whatever might be saved. Another example is the PSA test for prostate cancer—the test that the National Health Service wouldn't give me. Although there's debate as to the accuracy of the test for men of any age, almost all the experts agree that at a certain age—say, men who are over seventy years old—the test becomes counterproductive. If it shows signs of prostate cancer, the patient and his family may agitate for surgery to eliminate the cancer; but in men over seventy, that expensive intervention generally makes the patient's health worse and doesn't extend life expectancy (a seventy-year-old with prostate cancer is likely to die of something else before the cancer becomes dangerous). For that population of men, the "preventive" test doesn't prevent much and adds to the system's costs.

But as long as doctors and public health officials are judicious about which tests and procedures to use, the benefits of preventive care can be substantial. This is particularly true in advanced industrialized countries, where the major causes of premature death today are chronic diseases caused at least in part by diet, lifestyle, and tobacco use. The U.S. government says that nearly 40 percent of these early deaths are preventable. The cost of treating the chronic diseases—which can be a million dollars or more for one patient—is also preventable. So it benefits both the population and the health care system of any country to have a strong preventive medicine program in place.

As noted above, a unified health care system for everybody will have strong incentives to invest in preventive medicine. Britain's NHS, a single national system that cares for the entire population cradle to grave, seems to me to be the gold standard when it comes to preventive care. The British payment structure for general practitioners—the "capitation" system, which means a doctor gets paid by the number of patients on his list, and the pay-for-performance system, which gives the doctor extra income for keeping his patients healthy—drives the doctors to practice preventive care every day. But you don't have to go to the doctor's office to see NHS prevention at work. For one thing, the NHS has its own corps of "home health visitors," a large team of nurses who walk the streets and knock on doors to ask people if they have any concerns about their health. And then there's NHS Direct, a free phone line that anybody in the United Kingdom can call any day, anytime, to talk to a nurse about a medical problem. When we lived in London, I called NHS Direct a few times about some ailment in our family. The nurse would try to determine if a doctor was needed. If so, she would ask politely what time she should schedule the house call: "Tell me, love: Could the doctor come round about teatime?"

Everywhere you go in Britain, you are surrounded by brochures, posters, newspaper ads, radio announcements, and TV spots encouraging you—begging you, in fact—to guard your own health by taking advantage of a vast range of preventive services. All free, of course. Walking down the street in any British city, reading the NHS billboards, I used to get the impression that an army of well-trained, caring medical professionals was committed to the mission of keeping me healthy. The notices are everywhere, and they seem to cover almost everything:

You'll never regret an eye test. Get it free by calling 0845 766 9999.

Meningitis can kill!
Ring 020 8753 1081 to learn the symptoms.

Stop Smoking—We Can Help, for Free.
ring Stop Smoking, 020-8846-6840
or visit www.hf-pct.nhs.uk/quitsmoking

Manage Your Arthritis, Naturally. Freephone: 0800 652 3188

You can eat better! Visit www.wholegrain.co.uk

Management guidance for Dyspepsia.
Call the NHS Response Line, 0870 1555 455

Helping you to Better Sight
Please contact the Information Resources Team on 020 7278 1114

Aged 65 or over?

Make sure you get your pneumo jab.

Breathless?

British Lung Foundation Helpline: 08458 50 50 20

If You Knew About Flu, You'd Get the Jab

Are you concerned about food poisoning?

Contact the council's food safety team.

Take Care of Yourself

Get Your Free NHS Breast Screen

And then, when it is necessary to see a doctor, the NHS takes pains to make sure patients make the most of the visit. Each time our family went to our neighborhood surgery (doctor's office), we received an NHS flyer headlined "Questions to ask." It recommended that we ask the doctor things like: "Can I check that I've understood what you said?" "Can you write down any medical terms that I didn't understand?" "How and when will I get the test results?" "Who do I contact if I don't get the results?" "Who do I contact if things get worse?" The NHS also maintains a telephone hotline (free, of course) for people using medical equipment like blood pressure machines, syringes, hearing aids, and wheelchairs. "Faulty medical equipment?" the poster says. "Don't delay, report it today."

The British, like most other European countries, consider prenatal and postnatal care for a mother and her new child to be a central element of the preventive medicine routine. In this field, too, Britain's NHS is a leader. "As soon as the line turns blue" on the pregnancy test, the system kicks in with a broad range of services and benefits, including free prescriptions, home visits from a nurse and midwife, and a choice of birthing facilities. My friend Helen Ward had a baby on August 8, 2006, in the Whittington Hospital in North London. Helen is a reporter, and she kept detailed notes of her pregnancy.

I asked Helen how much she paid for the care she was provided at the doctor's office, at the hospital, and in her home. "Well, let's see," she said, consulting her notes. "When we had the sonogram, they make you pay £2 if you want a copy of the picture. And when labor began, we called a taxi to get to hospital. Well, you have to pay for the taxi; it's a tenner. So that's what it cost me to have a baby, I guess. Twelve quid. What would that come to in American money? Twenty dollars?"

And then Helen asked me a question: "My friends say that in America, you have to pay for antenatal visits, and delivery, and the postnatal. But that is hard for me to understand. Obviously, all that medical care is going to make sure the mother and the baby are healthy. Isn't that what a medical system is supposed to do? Keep people healthy, not let them get sick?

"So, could I just ask you: Why would you charge somebody to have a baby?"

It's a good question.

All the industrialized countries, except the United States, provide various other benefits for expectant mothers, such as free prescriptions, free dental care (because pregnant women and new mothers are unusually susceptible to tooth infection), free childbirth classes, and free nursing help at home in the baby's first weeks of life. In much of Europe, the government pays the mother (or father) a salary to stay home and raise the child for a period ranging from four months (France) to two years (Norway). In Finland, the government gives each expectant mother a free baby bed; it's delivered to the home by a nurse who talks over the basics of baby care while she sets up the crib. All the countries list this care and benefit system under the rubric "preventive medicine." It's an accurate label. Careful medical and nursing attention before and after birth tends to prevent the kind of neonatal health emergencies that are tragic for the new family and hugely expensive for the health care system. It is largely because of this extensive preventive intervention before and after birth that all the other wealthy countries report rates of infant mortality (that is, death within the first year of life) that are one-half or one-third as high as America's.

Whereas all other nations work from the time the line turns blue to introduce a healthy new patient into their health care system, the United States first attends to its poorest mothers and newborns in the hospital on delivery day. There's no economic incentive for the system to get involved earlier. Until we adopt a health care system that encourages it, preventive health care will remain largely inaccessible to far too many Americans.

TWELVE

The First Question

Let's conjure up a typical American town. We'll call this mythical town Wilburton and place it far up north in the Minnesota Iron Country, about twenty-five miles south of the Canadian border. And in this fictional town, let's imagine two fictional women, both forty-eight years old, both single mothers, both of them hardworking, decent people. By considering the circumstances of these two women, we will consider the question of inequalities in American life. In particular, we'll try to answer an important question: In a land where all are created equal, which inequalities are we willing to accept?

One of our fictional forty-eight-year-old mothers is Wendy Wilbur, the granddaughter of the industrialist for whom the town is named. She is the third-generation CEO of the family company, the Wilbur Iron Works. Wendy was born to privilege, but she has never been one to sit back on her good luck and relax; rather, she works long, trying days managing the company, mollifying the stockholders, and striving to protect the pay and benefits of the seven hundred people who earn their livelihood at the Wilbur factory. Like most American CEOs, she is well compensated for her hard work. Wendy makes about $2.6 million per year, not to mention a bucketful of benefits that include an executive health insurance plan and a driver who arrives at her mansion each morning to take her to work. Wendy lives in the tony Wilbur Heights neighborhood with her sixteen-year-old daughter, Mary. Mary is a bright and diligent honor student who is studying Chinese and analytic algebra at Wilburton Academy.

A half-dozen miles away, in a two-room apartment over a laundromat in downtown Wilburton, lives our other forty-eight-year-old single mother, Juanita Gonzalez. Juanita was born in Texas and came north as a child when her mother heard that there was work to be had in northern Minnesota. Juanita had to leave school at age fifteen to make money and help her mother; she has been working ever since. She cleans houses by day and irons shirts at the laundromat some evenings. She is a reliable and careful worker, so her customers pay her well, at least by the standards of domestic help. She brings in about $26,000 in a good year; this is not a high wage in the United States, but it is above the federally defined level of poverty for a family of two. Thus Juanita is ineligible for Medicaid or other health care programs that provide some coverage for those considered poor. What with gas prices and auto-repair costs, Juanita can't afford to drive to work. Rather, she stands on a jammed city bus each morning, clutching her mop and bucket, to ride out to the wealthy neighborhoods where she cleans. But for Juanita, all this hard work has a point: She is determined that her sixteen-year-old daughter, Maria, will stay in school and get the diploma that Juanita never earned. Maria, in fact, is a bright and diligent honor student at her school, Wilburton Central High. But the inner-city high school doesn't offer advanced math courses, and the only foreign language in its curriculum is Spanish, which Maria already knows.

There's one other thing these two forty-eight-year-old single

mothers have in common: Both Wendy and Juanita have recently contracted ovarian cancer.

In Wendy's case, she mentioned to a doctor—at the annual physical
exam that her corporate insurance plan provides—that she had been
feeling bloated and had intermittent pain in her pelvis. The doctor gave
Wendy a CA-125 blood test; the lab reported back that the results
suggested a malignancy. This finding prompted a routine series of diagnostic measures, including a transvaginal sonogram and a rectovaginal
pelvic examination. Those tests confirmed a cancerous growth. It was
a sobering diagnosis; but in twenty-first-century America, a malignant
tumor in the ovaries is a curable disease. Wendy was quickly scheduled
for the standard surgery in such cases, a state-of-the-art procedure called
"total hysterectomy with bilateral salpingo-oophorectomy," which
costs about $55,000. A gynecological oncologist removed her ovaries,
and the cancer with it. Wendy recovered completely. Thanks to the skill
of American doctors and the advances of American medical technology, Wendy can expect to live another four decades, cancer-free. She
will see her daughter graduate from high school and college, and spend
many happy hours playing with her grandchildren.

Juanita, too, had been feeling bloated recently, with intermittent
pains in her pelvic region. She worried about what that might mean.
But for a self-employed domestic worker who has no health insurance,
these symptoms did not suggest a visit to a doctor. The idea of paying
$400 for an annual physical is simply a nonstarter on Juanita's income;
in fact, just about any medical treatment would blow a hole in her
budget. Juanita's chances of obtaining a total hysterectomy with bilateral salpingo-oophorectomy are roughly equal to her chances of flying
to the moon on gossamer wings. Rather, she responded to the symptoms the way uninsured people in America generally handle medical
ailments: She did her best to ignore the pain and get on with life.
Juanita's undetected cancer spread gradually beyond her ovaries, and

the increasing pain eventually made it impossible for her to work. Finally, Maria persuaded her mother to go to the emergency room. Juanita was treated there for free. By then, though, the malignancy was too widespread to treat. Juanita was sent back home with a prescription for painkillers. If this woman could have seen a doctor when she first noticed the symptoms, if she had had access to the standard diagnostic and surgical procedures, she could have been cured, just as Wendy was. Instead, Juanita will die before she turns fifty, and leave her teenaged daughter an orphan.

Both Wendy and Juanita are Americans, a status that guarantees them equal access to certain basic rights. Although the corporate CEO is vastly richer than the self-employed domestic cleaner, Wendy and Juanita both get one vote in any election. They both have the right to free public education for their daughters. If these women were accused of a crime, both would have the right to the full panoply of legal protections in the courtroom. Both women have the same access to police protection, public libraries, state parks, trash pickup, and other services provided by government.

But many aspects of life in America, of course, are not equal for everybody. And hardly anybody suggests that all inequalities should be eliminated. A philosopher could presumably make the case that it is unfair for Wendy to make a salary one hundred times as large as Juanita's, since both women work equally long, hard days. The progressive income tax evens out that variance to a minor degree, but nobody is suggesting that society should insist that all wages be equalized. This is an inequality we tolerate. Similarly, it is probably wrong, in some cosmic sense of fairness, that one woman sits comfortably in a chauffeured limousine on the way to work each morning while the other stands on a crowded city bus, yet nobody is suggesting that society should provide a limousine for all morning commuters. This, too, is an inequality we tolerate. Many Americans chafe at the disparity in facilities and curriculum between penny-pinching inner-city high schools and the educational palaces erected a few miles away by well-endowed suburban school boards. But this is another inequality that our society tolerates, albeit with some mechanisms to even things out.

The final inequality, though, between Wendy's circumstance and Juanita's is downright lethal. One of these Wilburton women has access to the curative miracles of contemporary American medicine, and one does not. Because we have built a health care system that discriminates on the basis of wealth, the American health care system lets one woman live and the other die. Are we willing, as a society, to tolerate that inequality? The world's other developed countries have all considered that question, and all have answered: "No." As we've seen throughout this book, no other industrialized democratic country allows people to die from treatable diseases because they can't afford the doctor's bill. Indeed, if Juanita had lived about thirty miles farther north, just above the Canadian border, she would have had access to the same physical exams and the same doctor's care that Wendy received. In Canada, both of our single mothers would have been treated—although they might have waited longer than Wendy did to see a doctor—and both would have lived.

Would the recent changes to America's health care system have helped Juanita? Maybe. Under the 2010 reforms, Medicaid eligibility will be expanded. A broader Medicaid program might include a two-member family at Juanita's income level. And beginning in 2014, Juanita would be able to buy a private insurance policy for her family through a state "exchange"—that is, an insurance market—with tax credits from the federal government to help her pay the premium.

Wendy and Juanita are fictional Americans, created to illustrate a point. But Juanita's plight—death from a disease that could have been treated—is not a hypothetical case. It happens to tens of thousands of nonfiction Americans every year. The best-known study of this phenomenon is *Care Without Coverage: Too Little, Too Late,* published in 2002 by the Institute of Medicine, a branch of the National Academy of Sciences that advises Congress on health care trends and policy.[1] Despite its somewhat dramatic title, *Care Without Coverage* is a dry, technical 193-page research report that draws on two lengthy census studies to measure the impact of not having health insurance. After extensive analysis, the report arrives at the key equation:

$$DT = DI + DU = (PI \times n) + (PU \times 1.25)$$

Basically, this formula says that People who are Uninsured (PU) are 25 percent more likely to die of treatable diseases than People of the same age cohort who have Insurance (PI). Adding up the additional deaths in each ten-year group between the ages of twenty-five and sixty-four, the Institute of Medicine concluded that 18,314 Americans die each year because they don't have health insurance and thus can't get the treatment that would save their lives. By age group, the study concluded that some 2,000 Americans between twenty-five and thirty-four die each year from lack of access to health care. This grim statistic increases for each ten-year cohort; in the age group from fifty-five to sixty-four, 8,200 Americans die annually because they can't afford health care. (Starting at age sixty-five, uninsured Americans have Medicare coverage, and thus they generally get the treatment they need.)

The Institute of Medicine based its finding on data from the year 2000, when there were roughly 30 million Americans without health insurance. By 2009, there were some 45 million Americans who spent at least part of the year without health coverage. Applying the institute's formula to updated statistics, the Urban Institute increased the estimate. This updated estimate suggests that more than 22,000 Americans are left to die each year because they can't afford medical care.[2] Another 2009 study at Harvard Medical School, using a somewhat modified formula, said that "as many as 44,789 deaths per year" among Americans are due to lack of health coverage.[3]

The Institute of Medicine study said that people without insurance are more likely to die both from disease and from accidents. Uninsured people who are hit by automobiles in the United States routinely get less trauma care than those with insurance and are 37 percent more likely to die, even if their injuries are normal and treatable. Uninsured people with various cancers are 30 to 50 percent more likely to die, the report said. This is largely because people without insurance don't get the tests and screenings that tend to detect cancer early enough for effective treatment. "When cancer is found, it is relatively advanced and more often fatal than it is in persons with health insurance coverage," the study said. The same is true for chronic illnesses like diabetes, hypertension, cardiac disease, and lupus. Because they don't have access to diagnostic tests and don't see a doctor when the early symptoms appear, American adults without insurance tend to die by the thousands each year from these diseases, even though effective treatments exist.

The Americans who suffer and die are not, for the most part, homeless or addicted or desperately poor. Most of those who die for lack of medical treatment in the world's richest country are working Americans who run afoul of the nation's complicated and restrictive health insurance labyrinth, both public and private.

The late Monique "Nikki" White, the bright, vivacious young woman we met on the first page of this book, was one such American. Unlike the two women of Wilburton, Nikki was a real person, and her story is tragically nonfiction. Tall, slender, athletic, she grew up in a middle-class family in Bristol, Tennessee; her parents were both middle managers in corporate America, and she was covered by a family health insurance plan until she finished college in 1999. She earned a degree in psychology at the University of Texas and went to work after college for a bookstore near the campus in Austin. It was a perfect job for her. But Nikki, beginning to feel ill, felt obliged to look for a job with health benefits—the bookstore didn't provide them, and her parents' plan wouldn't cover her after she finished school. She found work at a hospital in Austin, where she was eligible for the employee health insurance plan. Some days, Nikki was too sick to go to work; she developed severe stomach pains, extreme fatigue, and skin lesions on various parts of her body. A doctor confirmed that Nikki had contracted systemic lupus erythematosus, a chronic inflammatory disease that mainly strikes women. This was not good news, but it was hardly a death sentence; about 80 percent of Americans with lupus live a normal life span. "For the vast majority of people with lupus," says the Lupus Foundation of America, "effective treatment can minimize symptoms, reduce inflammation, and maintain normal bodily functions."[4] But effective treatment requires health insurance.

In 2001, Nikki was so ill that she had to leave work. That's when the long, frustrating, and eventually fatal struggle with America's health care system began for Nikki White. Like most working Americans, she lost her health insurance when she lost her job. "The timing was just tragic," said her family physician, Dr. Amylyn Crawford. "The insurance system dropped her at the point when she needed it most." With grim determination, Nikki applied to every individual insurance plan she could find—in vain. No for-profit insurance company in the United States was willing to cover a person who had chronic lupus. Unemployed and uninsured, she moved home and set up an apartment over her mother's garage in the green, rolling Appalachian country where Tennessee, North Carolina, and Virginia meet. This not only provided free housing, but the return to Tennessee also meant she could enroll in TennCare, the local version of Medicaid, the government program that provides health insurance for the poorest Americans. Nikki had trouble finding a specialist who would treat her condition at Medicaid's payment rates—Medicaid pays doctors less than Medicare, the U.S. government program for the elderly—but eventually she found a rheumatologist who agreed to take her on. The doctor prescribed azathiopine, a drug that would control the inflammation that was causing painful lesions on Nikki's chest and hands. He warned her clearly that this powerful medication could have dangerous side effects. To avoid them, she needed regular blood tests, CT scans, and office checkups. Neither Nikki nor her mother could pay for such expensive care. Fortunately, they had TennCare to help.

In the summer of 2005, though, Tennessee cut back sharply on its TennCare insurance program. Under the new rules, Nikki White had too much money to qualify for Medicaid. Once again, she was uninsured. She kept trying to get health coverage, but all her appeals were denied. By now, her hands were so painful from the lesions that she had to wear thick gloves just to fill out an application. "She fought and she fought and she fought," Dr. Crawford recalled later. For months at a time, as Nikki dealt with a bewildering onslaught of cold bureaucratic form letters, it was unclear whether she was insured or not. "If your TennCare has ended, you should not have gotten this letter," one missive said. That was followed by another, equally mysterious: "If this box is checked, the person listed in line 3 has at least 18 months creditable coverage. IMPORTANT! This does not mean you have coverage now." The state Department of Human Services sent TennCare Form Letter 207.5, explaining the extent of her legal right to get insurance: "You can still apply for individual health insurance coverage. Some companies **may** let you buy a different kind of insurance (*not* a HIPAA plan). But, they **don't** have to. AND, they **don't** have to cover pre-existing conditions."

Nikki White was a college graduate and had worked in medical care. She knew how to research health insurance regulations. Eventually, she figured out that Medicaid would have to give her coverage if she was legally determined to be "disabled." She began filing applications with yet another government department, the Social Security Administration, the agency that determines whether or not an American is disabled. Denied. By the summer of 2005, Nikki White began to fear that she would never get the medical care she needed. "I don't want to die," she said on her thirty-second birthday. "Please don't let me die."

In her last weeks of life, Nikki began to receive medical care. In November of 2005, she suffered a seizure—due to kidney failure and perforated intestine—and was admitted to the emergency ward at Bristol Regional Medical Center. From that point on, her insurance problems didn't matter; under federal law, the hospital had to treat her until her condition was "stable." Over ten weeks, she had more than twenty-five operations, all provided gratis. By then, though, the patient was too sick for any hospital to save. In the spring of 2006, at the age of thirty-two, Nikki White died. Officially, the cause of death was listed as "complications of lupus." In fact, as her doctor said, the proximate cause of death was a health care system that failed to provide the treatment that would have saved her life.

Monique White was an American citizen, guaranteed equal access, along with every other American, to certain basic rights. But she didn't have equal access to health care. If Nikki had received the standard treatment regimen for lupus readily available to any American with health insurance, she could have lived a normal life span. If she had been a resident of any other developed nation, she could have lived a normal life span. No other rich country would have tolerated the inequality that left Nikki White dead.

Which inequalities will society tolerate? Is it acceptable that some people are left to die because they can't see a doctor when they get sick? That question encompasses a more basic question: Is health care a human right?

Should society guarantee health care, the way we guarantee the right to think and pray as you like, to get an education, to vote in free elections? Or is medicine a commodity to be bought and sold, a product like a car, a computer, or a camera? This is the key question facing any nation as it designs a health care system. Professor William Hsiao, the Harvard economist, has helped design health care systems for more than a dozen nations. He says the creation of a national health care system involves political, economic, and medical decisions, but the primary decision to be made is a moral one.

"Before you can set up a health care system for any country," Hsiao told me, "you have to know that country's basic ethical values. The first question is: Do people in your country have a right to health care? If the people believe that medical care is a basic right, you design a system that means anybody who is sick can see a doctor. If a society considers medical care to be an economic commodity, then you set up a system that distributes health care based on the ability to pay. And then the poor, pretty much, are left out." Hsiao referred to this fundamental choice as a matter of "distributional ethics." "Your ethics, your sense of justice, determine how you distribute goods and services, including health care," Hsiao said. "So the first question has to deal with a country's ethical values."

If your notion of "distributional ethics" tells you that health care is an area of human life in which everyone should be treated the same, then you would design a system like the ones I saw in Canada, or Germany, or Japan, where the rich and the poor have equal access to the same doctors and the same drugs. You would look at health care the way the physician we met in chapter 4, Dr. Valerie Biousse, described the French view: "When we get sick, then everybody is equal." On the other hand, if you believe that the most important national goals are economic prosperity, good jobs for all, and financial rewards for entrepreneurs who take risks to create wealth and jobs, then you might design a health care system like the one the United States has today, where the well-off get the best medical care in the world, and people in the bottom brackets get so little care that thousands die of treatable diseases.

All the developed countries except the United States have decided that every human has a basic right to health care. Many international organizations have reached the same conclusion. When distinguished commissions of scholars and government officials from around the world get together to produce some flowery—but essentially unenforceable—declaration on "the rights of man," they almost always include language that includes a "fundamental right" to some level of health care.

In 1948, when the members of the newly formed United Nations decided to enunciate a global consensus on basic human rights, their Universal Declaration of Human Rights included the assurance that "everyone has the right to a standard of living adequate for the health and well-being of himself and of his family, including food, clothing, housing and medical care."[5] Two decades later, the UN's 1966 International Covenant on Economic, Social, and Cultural Rights decreed that every nation is responsible for "the creation of conditions which would assure, to all, medical service and medical attention in the event of sickness."[6] Numerous other groupings of countries have reached similar conclusions, including the European Union, the Pan-American Union, and the World Health Organization.

All those high-minded declarations may have some inspirational or political value, but a piece of paper issued by an international organization rarely conveys a "right" that has practical value. (In fact, the United States has signed most of those international pronouncements, but has never implemented a universal right to health care within its own borders.) A legal right has more practical impact when it is offered by a national or regional government. Most European nations have recognized a right to health care for everyone, either in the national constitution or in statutory law. And these declarations have made a difference. In the heady days after World War II, the new democratic government of Italy put forth a Constitution that included a Bill of Rights designed to be a clear statement of the rights that Italians were denied under the Fascists. Among many other guarantees, the Italian Constitution pledges that "the Republic protects health as a fundamental right of the individual and as a concern of the collective state, and guarantees free care to the indigent." At the time, it was mere rhetoric; Italy had no system in place to make that "fundamental right of the individual" a reality. But in 1978, when the *Parlamento* got around to creating a national health care system, the members opted for a national health service plan on the Beveridge Model.[7]

Today, nearly all European nations (Russia is the striking exception) recognize the Charter of Fundamental Rights of the European Union, a legal declaration that acts as a common Bill of Rights for the twenty-seven member states of the E.U. This expansive document includes all the protections set forth in the U.S. Bill of Rights (except the right to own a gun). But then it goes far beyond the U.S. Constitution, granting every European the right to a paid vacation, the right to strike, the right to paid parental leave when a baby is born, the right to a clean environment, the right to "a high level of consumer protection," and even "the right of access to a free placement service" when looking for a job. Given that laundry list, it's hardly surprising that the European Charter also includes a right to health care:

> Everyone has the right of access to preventive health care and the right
> to benefit from medical treatment under the conditions established by
> national laws and practices. A high level of human health protection
> shall be ensured in the definition and implementation of all Union
> policies and activities.[8]

About thirty nations around the world have written new constitutions in recent decades, a rush that was largely propelled by the boom in newly independent countries following the collapse of the Soviet Union. Nearly all of them have included a right to health care. The Czech Republic, for example, revamped its constitution in 1992 and added a lengthy bill of rights that says, "The state is obliged to guarantee the right to life and the right to protection of health and health care for all."[9]

BUT ONCE A NATION HAS DECLARED, as a legal matter, that everybody has a right to health care, how do you enforce the right? Is it a "justiciable" right—that is, something that courts will enforce? If you show up at some doctor's door, is she required to treat you, because you have a fundamental human right to treatment? For the most part, the developed nations that legally declare a right to health care have implemented that right not by imposing duties on particular doctors or hospitals but, rather, by setting up some national system of care that is available to everybody, regardless of wealth. As we've seen in this book, the basic principle that everyone should have access to medical care doesn't dictate how a national system will work. Some countries agree with the Italian view that if there's a right to care, the government is required to create facilities that provide care. Others have concluded that the private sector and private insurance can meet the need, with the crucial proviso that the insurance system has to cover everybody (even those with a chronic case of lupus); as a corollary, these countries require as well that everybody buy insurance, to give the insurance plans a broad enough risk pool to keep them solvent.

In most countries, though not the United States, the existence of a legal right to health care has generated a good deal of litigation, generally filed by plaintiffs who say they didn't get the care they were entitled to. Generally, these plaintiffs lose. The courts, for the most part, have accepted each country's health care system as it is. As we saw in chapter 7, there have been cases in Britain where sick people, invoking their right to health care, have gone to court to force the National Health Service to provide a particular drug or procedure or prosthetic device that is not covered. The judges routinely side with the NHS. The courts have concluded that the national system—or its rationing body, NICE—can set the rules for prescriptions and treatment, as long as everybody has equal access to the care that is provided.

Similarly, the highest court in Taiwan ruled in 2002 that everyone in the country has a right to health care, but that it is the job of the Bureau of National Health Insurance to determine which medicines and medical procedures are included in that right.

Citizens of the United States have lots of rights, some guaranteed by the Constitution, some provided by statute, some created and protected by the courts. But the U.S. Constitution does not guarantee a right to health care. None of the fifty state constitutions does, either. Occasionally some American goes to court asserting that there is a right to medical treatment; generally, the legal claim is predicated on the notion that all men have certain inalienable rights, according to our Declaration of Independence, and that among these is the right to life, and that you can't have life without medical care to keep you alive. No American court has ever bought this argument. Some legal scholars note, acerbically, that the only Americans with a legal right to demand medical care are prisoners; there have been cases where judges have ordered prisons to provide medical treatment for an ailing inmate. The prisoners appreciate it. A twenty-year-old inmate named Melissa Matthews in Tacoma, Washington, declined parole and chose to stay in jail because she had cervical cancer. "If I'm in here, then I can get treated," Matthews told KING-TV. "If I'm out, I'm going to die from this cancer."[10] For the law-abiding, health care in the United States is a product, something that Americans are expected to buy if they can afford it. If you are a senior, a soldier, a veteran, a Native American, a member of Congress, or a renal-failure victim, or if you are scratching by on an income below the designated rate of poverty, government will help you obtain health care. All the rest—that is, about 70 percent of the population—are on their own.

Under the health reform law passed in 2010, the number of Americans with health insurance will be significantly increased. But even when that law takes full effect, roughly 23 million people will still be uninsured—and thus no better off than Nikki White.

WHY DOESN'T THE UNITED STATES recognize a right to medical care? Are Americans so cold, so callous, so obsessed with their own lives and bank accounts that they don't care if their neighbors can't afford to see a doctor? The answer is: No. In fact, when pollsters ask the basic question—"Do you think everybody has a right to medical care when they get sick?"—more than 85 percent of Americans answer that health care is a basic human right. And yet our nation does not provide it. The result is that the world's richest nation allows twenty-two thousand of its people to die each year from treatable diseases.

One reason our society lets this happen is that most Americans don't know that it's happening. Americans generally believe that anybody who needs health care in the United States can get it, either through health insurance or charity. Opinion polls frequently ask questions designed to gauge public awareness of the plight of the uninsured. A common formulation is "Do you think people in your community, rich or poor, can get the medical care they need when they get sick?" To this question, roughly nine out of ten Americans answer "Yes." They may not know the exact mechanism for getting care to the uninsured, but most Americans believe our society provides it. President George W. Bush repeatedly assured the American people that they need not worry about their uninsured neighbors. "I mean, people have access to health care in America," Bush told a business meeting in Cleveland on July 10, 2007. "After all, you just go to the emergency room."[11]

But the president was wrong. As a rule, you can't just go to the emergency room in America unless you have the cash or the insurance coverage to pay the bill. Hospitals routinely turn sick people away if they can't prove they have the means to pay. This is legal. "A hospital is not, as a general rule, required to provide non-emergency care to persons unable to pay," notes the leading U.S. Textbook on the law of health care. "It is also not required to continue treatment in the face of nonpayment of bills."[12] In the 1980s, there were several well-publicized cases, sometimes caught on videotape, of patients who were "dumped" onto the streets in their hospital robes because they couldn't pay. The resulting uproar led Congress to pass the Emergency Medical Treatment and Active Labor Act of 1986—a statute known by its acronym, EMTALA, or by its popular name, the Patient Anti-Dumping Act. Under EMTALA, any hospital receiving Medicare funds has to admit and treat anybody who is (1) facing severe risk of death, or (2) in active labor, until the patient's medical condition is "stabilized." (After Bush's comment in Cleveland the White House explained that EMTALA was what the president had in mind.) Because of this legal requirement, and because there's a culture of public service in the hospital industry, American hospitals provide care each year to millions of acutely ill or injured patients who can't pay their bills. But most sick people aren't on the verge of death or in the final stages of childbirth, so most of the time EMTALA doesn't help at all. The reality is that you can't "just go the emergency room" for the physical exam or the blood test or the breast palpation that could diagnose a disease before it threatens your life. You can't just go to the ER to refill the prescription for the pills that would keep you alive. As Nikki White learned, you can't just go to the emergency room for regular examinations and CT scans to guard against the side effects of azathiopine.

Beyond this general ignorance about the fate of the uninsured, Americans have never really carried on an ethical debate about health care as a right—that is, about which inequalities we are willing to tolerate. The U.S. health care system developed without much planning, and without the serious assessment of national values that prompted other nations to create systems for universal care. As we saw in chapter 10, President Clinton presented his health-care-for-all plan in 1993 not as a moral obligation but, rather, as an economic initiative: "Reforming health care is essential to reducing the deficit and expanding investment."[13] During the long and sometimes ferocious argument over "Obamacare," a nation's moral obligation to provide health care for all was barely mentioned. President Obama himself spent months talking mainly about economic concerns; only in the final weeks before the decisive Congressional votes did he focus on the plight of the uninsured. Opponents of the bill complained about deficit spending and a "government takeover" of medicine. Neither the president nor his critics found it politically useful to discuss the value of covering everybody, since neither side was pushing that idea. The ethical issue of universal coverage—Professor Hsiao's "first question"—was not part of the conversation. It has never been part of the conversation in the United States.

But some Americans have been pressing their countrymen to deal with that "first question" as a foundation for building a new national health care system. Professor Uwe Reinhardt, the economist at Princeton University and global leader in the field of health care economics, argues that U.S. policy makers have deliberately avoided the moral question. "Typically," Reinhardt says, "the opponents of universal health insurance cloak their sentiments in actuarial technicalities or in the mellifluous language of the standard economic theory of markets, thereby avoiding a debate on ideology that truly might engage the American public."[14]

In 1997, to ignite a debate on the moral basis of American health care, Reinhardt wrote an article for the nation's leading medical journal, the *Journal of the American Medical Association,* posing a simple question: If the child of a rich American family and the child of a poor American family both contract the same illness, should both children have the same chance at being cured?

Judging from opinion polls, most Americans, and indeed most doctors, would probably answer "Yes" to that question. But the responses that came in to the AMA journal were uniformly negative. "Professor Reinhardt is resorting to the effete ploy of class warfare," thundered one physician. "Professor Reinhardt's pointed question is . . . socialist propaganda," wrote another, "a loaded question complete with the ancient propagandistic use of children." Professor Richard Epstein, of the University of Chicago Law School, offered a direct reply to Reinhardt's question as to whether the rich and the poor should have the same chance to get medical care: "The correct answer is no," Epstein wrote. To provide health care for the poor child, he argued, other Americans would have to be taxed to pay for the care. That would generate heated and costly political battles. "To open the doors to forced redistribution induces the rich to spend more defending their wealth, and the poor to spend more to take it away. Both sides cannot win, and a smaller pie leads to worse health care."[15]

Obviously the cost of health care could shoot upward toward infinite levels if everybody had the right to the full range of testing, treatment, surgery, and medication afforded by state-of-the-art contemporary medicine. To offer all possible treatment to every patient would lead any health care system rapidly toward bankruptcy. For this reason, other developed nations have framed the right to universal health care in terms of a floor and a ceiling. There is some floor level of care—that is, the basic package of benefits—to which everybody has access. Generally, this includes standard diagnostics and treatment for disease, some level of preventive care, and access, either for free or a small fee, to an approved list of drugs. And there is generally a ceiling beyond which the system will not go. Some expensive drugs, some advanced surgical interventions, cosmetic surgery, and so on will generally not be covered by the health care system. Some effective but expensive procedures will not be covered for a patient who has only a brief time left to live. Some nations—including Canada, as we saw in chapter 8—have tried to make it illegal for people to buy health care that is above the ceiling by denying doctors and hospitals the right to perform any procedure that is not on the approved list. But these efforts to limit what rich people can buy almost always fail. A wealthy patient who is denied care in his own country is likely to cross the border and pay a doctor in the nation next door. Accordingly, the developed nations maintain a floor of basic coverage available to everyone, and a ceiling on the treatments the national system will pay for. As we saw earlier in this book, the former British health minister John Reid put it succinctly: "We cover everybody, but we don't cover everything."

The United States differs from all the other developed nations in that it has no floor and no ceiling. For tens of millions of people, the American health care system offers little or no care (or no care until it is too late, as in the case of Nikki White). For people covered by top-of-the-line insurance plans, the U.S. system offers almost anything, regardless of the price or the patient's age.

If the people of the United States were to resolve the ethical question—if we were to decide, for example, that all Americans should have access to a doctor when they're sick—we would still have many questions to answer. Once a nation recognizes a fundamental right to some adequate level of health care, it still has to define what is "adequate." Which drugs and treatments should be available; which should be left out of the basic package? If the goal is "equity," what is an equitable method of financing health care? Should everyone pay an equal amount, in taxes or insurance premiums? Should older people or sick people pay more because they tend to use more care? Or should we tell the young and the healthy that they are lucky to have youth and health and should be willing to subsidize the care of those who aren't so lucky? Does a right to health care mean the same thing as a "right to health"? Does "equity" mean that a nation should have a standard health care system that cares for everybody—or can we maintain our separate systems for veterans, for seniors, for congressmen?

Before we get to problems like that, though, the United States will have to face William Hsiao's "first question." What are our basic ethical values? Do we believe that every American has a right to health care when he needs it? After that question is resolved, we can move on to the task of designing a health care system that works for all Americans. When we get to that stage, we can draw on a world of ideas and experience—all the lessons we've learned from health care systems in the other industrialized democracies.

THIRTEEN

Major Surgery

I SET OUT ON MY GLOBAL QUEST LOOKING FOR SOLUTIONS to two nagging medical complaints. One was a personal concern, something that matters only to me: a cure for my ailing right shoulder. The other was a major national issue that matters to all 304 million Americans: a cure for our nation's ailing, unfair, and absurdly expensive health care system. By the end of my medical odyssey, after a dozen countries and several dozen doctors, I felt successful on both points. I didn't find a miracle cure in either case. But I came away confident that solutions are at hand. My stiff shoulder is looser today and considerably less painful than when I set out. More important, I found fundamental operating principles overseas that would help the United States provide quality health care to everybody and save money in the process. The fact is, we can fix the basic problems facing American health care—cost, coverage, and quality—if we're willing to copy some of the ideas that have worked in other wealthy industrialized democracies around the world.

As I TRAVELED from one nation's orthopedic specialist to the next, I came to realize a key point: Major surgery was "not indicated," as the doctors say, for my shoulder. The total shoulder arthroplasty, or replacement, that my American doctor recommended probably would have produced a good result, but at a formidable cost: serious pain, months of rehabilitation, and tens of thousands of dollars. In the course of my global tour, other doctors showed me that there were other treatments for my particular problem, less drastic and less expensive. In Japan, Dr. Nakamichi suggested that periodic steroid injections could alleviate the pain I had been accustomed to feeling for years when I rolled over onto my right shoulder. That seems to have worked; I don't wake up with a wince anymore. In France, Dr. Tamalet prescribed regular physical therapy at a spa (in France, of course, such delights are covered by health insurance). That was clearly sound advice, because the spa-style therapeutic massage I received under Dr. Manohar's care at the *chikitsalayam* in India led to significant improvement. In Taiwan, Dr. Li Mei-Li gave me acupuncture treatment; it didn't help a bit, but it didn't hurt much either, so it was certainly worth a try. Surprisingly, Dr. Badat, in London, made a useful contribution, too, even as he was telling me that the National Health Service wouldn't spend a penny to fix my stiff shoulder. "Just learn to live with it, mate," the blunt Dr. Badat said, in a tone that suggested he gives this advice to a lot of his patients. Somehow, this stoic dictate has indeed helped me to live with it.

My world of treatment has had a positive outcome: My shoulder is better. I still can't swing a golf club and probably never will again; I've learned to live with that. Still, the daily pain has pretty much disappeared, and my range of motion has definitely increased. And I got that outcome without major surgery; I didn't really need a total shoulder replacement.

AMERICA'S HEALTH CARE SYSTEM, in contrast, does require major surgery. My global quest demonstrated that America's approach to health care is unique in the world for a good reason: No other country would dream of doing things the way we do. So it's clear that we can't fix the basic problems by tinkering at the margins of our existing system. Any proposal for "reform" that continues to rely on our fragmented structure of overlapping and often conflicting payment systems for different subsets of the population will not reduce the cost or the complexity of American health care. Any proposal that sticks with our current dependence on for-profit private insurers—corporations that pick and choose the people they want to cover and the claims they want to pay—will not be sustainable. The health care reform bill that Congress passed in 2010 made significant changes in the existing U.S. health care system. (For a description of that bill, see the afterword of this book.) If the law works as planned, it will substantially increase the number of people with health insurance. It outlaws some of the crueler practices of the American health insurance industry. It has mechanisms that might slow the increase in health care costs. But the law does nothing to simplify the "crazy quilt" structure of different systems for different population groups; if anything, American health care will be even more complicated and difficult to navigate when "Obamacare" takes full effect. And the new law will not get us to universal coverage, the bedrock principle of health care systems in every other industrialized democracy.

So major surgery is still indicated. And yet the United States does not need a total system replacement. Some elements of our health care infrastructure are working well—particularly the education and training of doctors, nurses, technicians, and so on, and our state-of-the-art medical research, where America leads the world.

To put it simply, the United States does well when it comes to providing medical care, but has a rotten system for financing that care. We need a health care system that permits the strong facets of American medicine to flourish, makes their benefits accessible to everybody, and does it in a cost-efficient way. As we've seen, this is not impossible. All the other rich countries have found financing mechanisms that cover everybody and they still spend much less than we do. We've ignored those foreign models, partly because of "American exceptionalism"—the notion that the United States has nothing to learn from the rest of the world. In health care, at least, that old mindset is clearly losing its sway. Americans are coming to realize that the other rich countries are getting more and better medicine, for less money, than we do.

Another reason Americans tend to ignore the valuable lessons we could take from the rest of the world is that we have been in thrall to conventional wisdom about health care overseas. Thus we conclude that the foreign approaches would never work here. In fact, as I found on my global quest, much of this conventional wisdom is wrong. A lot of what we "know" about other nations' approach to health care is simply myth. To summarize what we've seen in this book, here are five common American myths about health care systems overseas:

MYTH 1: "IT'S ALL SOCIALIZED MEDICINE OUT THERE."

This venerable notion has become such a commonplace in the United States that it transcends our nation's political divide. Conservative think tanks and presidential candidates routinely declare that "European-style socialized medicine" cannot work in the capitalistic USA. On the left, producer Michael Moore made the same assumption in his satirical documentary *Sicko*—except Moore argued that foreign medical systems work better than ours because they're all "socialized." In fact, it's not all socialized medicine out there. Most wealthy countries rely on private-sector mechanisms to provide and/or pay for health care. Indeed, some foreign health care systems are more privatized than ours.

As we've seen, the Beveridge Model countries (such as Britain, Spain, Italy, Cuba) do provide health care in government hospitals, with government paying the bills. This model, with government serving as both provider and payer, probably comes closest to the concept of socialized medicine that Americans have in mind. But even the Beveridge system isn't fully socialist. The GPs in Britain, who provide most of the care, are private businesspeople—and they can be ferocious capitalists, like my stout, prosperous physician, Dr. Badat. The National Health Insurance countries (e.g., Canada, Taiwan) rely on private-sector doctors, hospitals, and labs but pay for their services through a government insurance plan. Public payment of private providers—should we call that semi-socialized medicine? The Bismarck Model countries (such as France, Germany, the Netherlands, Switzerland, Japan) offer universal coverage using private providers and private insurance plans—with government exercising various degrees of regulatory control over insurance coverage, pricing, and so on. Private-sector providers and private financing—it's hard to call that "socialized." In some aspects, "European-style" medicine is less socialized than America's. Almost all Americans take up government-run health care—Medicare—when they turn sixty-five. But as we've seen, people in Germany, Switzerland, and elsewhere stick with private insurance plans for life. In those countries, moreover, military veterans are covered by the same private insurance plans as everybody else. Meanwhile, the U.S. Department of Veterans Affairs operates one of the planet's purest examples of socialized medicine.

MYTH 2: "THEY RATION CARE WITH WAITING LISTS AND LIMITED CHOICE."

This common impression, too, runs counter to the facts. In many developed countries, people have quicker access to care and more choice than Americans do.

Germans can sign up for any of the nation's two hundred-plus private health insurance plans, a broader choice than any American has. If a German doesn't like her insurance company, she can switch to another, with no increase in premium. The Swiss, too, can choose any insurance plan in the country.

In France and Japan, you don't get a choice of insurance company; you have to use the one designated for your company or your municipality. But you do get total choice of providers; patients can go to any doctor, any hospital, any traditional healer in the entire country. There are no American-style limits like an "in-network" list of doctors, or "preauthorization" by the insurance company. Every provider in the country is in-network and authorized. You pick the doctor, the hospital, the lab, or the spa of your choice, and insurance has to pay. Canadians, similarly, have to pay into the government-run insurance plan for their province—no choice about that—but they can choose any doctor anywhere, and insurance will pay the bill.

As for those notorious waiting lists, some countries are plagued by them. As we've seen in this book, Canada and Britain limit the number of specialists and operating rooms in the system to save money, with the result that patients wait weeks or months for nonemergency care. But other nations—Germany, France, Sweden, Denmark— perform better than the United States on standard measures such as "Waiting time to see a specialist" and "Waiting time for elective surgery." As we saw in chapter 6, waiting times in Japan are so short that most patients don't bother to make an appointment. A fellow with a sore right shoulder can walk into Keio Daigaku Hospital and see the nation's top orthopedic surgeon on the same day; no appointment required.

MYTH 3: "THEY ARE WASTEFUL SYSTEMS RUN BY BLOATED BUREAUCRACIES."

It seems natural to Americans that free enterprise and profit-driven markets are the most efficient way to provide goods and services. So it's not surprising that Americans generally believe that that U.S.-style medicine—private-sector providers, financed by for-profit insurance—must be the most efficient way to provide health care. But this, too, turns out to be a myth. All the others systems in the developed world, public and private, are more frugal than ours.

America's for-profit health insurance companies have the highest administrative costs in the world. This is a major reason why we spend more for health care—and get less in return—than any other developed country. As we've seen, the estimates vary somewhat, but America's health insurance industry spends roughly 20 cents of every dollar for nonmedical costs: paperwork, reviewing claims, marketing, profits, and so on. France's private, but nonprofit, health insurance industry, in contrast, covers everybody but spends about 5 percent for administration. Canada's universal insurance system, run by government bureaucrats, spends 6 percent on administration. As we learned in chapter 10, Taiwan adopted a leaner version of Canada's National Health Insurance model for its national system. Taiwan's government-run financing system has administrative costs under 2 percent.

The world champion at controlling medical costs is Japan, even though its aging population is a profligate consumer of medical care. But those tough cost controls—like a bed in Dr. Kono's hospital for $15 per night—have not impaired the availability or the quality of care. The Japanese system has produced fantastic results: the longest-lived and healthiest population in the world. Yet the Japanese system is far more efficient than ours, spending less than half as much money per capita.

MYTH 4: "HEALTH INSURANCE COMPANIES HAVE TO BE CRUEL."

Americans tend to expect nasty treatment from health insurance companies, because that's what Americans get. Our insurance companies are mainly profit-making enterprises. They enhance their profits not by paying for people's health care, but by finding ways not to pay. They employ armies of adjusters to deny claims. When they accept a claim, the payment routinely takes weeks or months to arrive. It's no wonder Americans are the world's least satisfied health insurance customers. Insurance companies in the United States defend their tough business practices by noting that they're in a tough line of business. If they paid every claim in a timely fashion, they'd go broke.

But my trip around the world demonstrated that this, too, is a myth. In foreign health insurance systems—for example, those of France, Germany, Japan, and Switzerland—insurers have to accept all applicants, regardless of any previous diseases or accidents. They can't cancel coverage as long as you pay your premiums. They are required to pay any claim submitted by a doctor or hospital (or health spa), usually within tight time limits. The corollary is that everyone is mandated to buy insurance, to give the plans an adequate pool of rate payers. And with a large enough risk pool, these plans don't go broke. As we saw in Switzerland, the private health insurance companies are doing just fine, thank you, under these rules.

MYTH 5: "THOSE SYSTEMS ARE TOO FOREIGN TO WORK IN THE USA."

I encountered numerous approaches to providing and paying for health care in the course of my global quest. But each of them fell into one of the four basic categories set forth in chapter 2. Far from being "foreign," each of these systems is in use today in the United States. For veterans, active-duty military personnel, and Native Americans, we use the British model. For people over sixty-five, we've adopted the Canadian model (we even use the name for it that was coined by the socialist who invented the Canadian system: Medicare). For working people who get insurance through their employers, we're a Bismarck country, like Germany or Japan. And for the tens of millions without insurance coverage, we're just another Out-of-Pocket country. Of course the foreign models could work for Americans; they already do.

PERHAPS THE GREATEST MISCONCEPTION we have about foreign health care systems is that they're all the same. In fact, there are countless variations, large and small, in the way different nations organize the financing and delivery of health care. Some systems require a co-pay for any medical service, and others have no co-pays at all. Some offer free annual physical exams for everybody, and some don't. Most provide free medical care to expectant mothers and their newborn children, but Japanese health insurance doesn't cover pregnancy and childbirth (rather, the local government generally puts up the money for the medical expenses of mother and child). Even countries that share the same basic model manage specific issues in different ways. Some of the Bismarck Model countries (e.g., Germany, France) have a uniform health insurance premium pegged as a percentage of income, while others (e.g., Switzerland) let the insurance plans set their own premium rates.

Still, there are some standard building blocks of health care system architecture that all developed countries (except, of course, the United States) have agreed on. By studying the blueprints and looking at these common principles, we can learn some important lessons about fixing the problems in our own health care system.

A UNIFIED SYSTEM

All the other developed countries have decided to use one system of health care that applies to everybody. Young or old, employed or unemployed, military or civilian, sick or well, aboriginal or immigrant, private citizen or prime minister, newborn or about-to-die—everybody is included in the same system and covered by a single set of rules. All other rich nations have embraced this basic principle, because they think it's fairer if everybody in the country has the same access to the same level of care. They find a single system is much easier to administer, with one set of forms to fill out, one book of rules, and one price list. As an economic principle, a unified system is a powerful force for cost control. Since the single health care system is the only buyer of medical services, it has enormous market clout in negotiating fees with doctors, hospitals, drug companies, and so on. That's why an MRI scan that costs $1,200 in Denver is priced at $98 in Tokyo. That's why a pill that costs $1.20 in

Denver is priced at 20 cents in London. The doctors and drug companies don't like that meager price regime, but it's all they can get from their only source of payment.

A unified health care system that works the same for everybody doesn't necessarily equate to a single-payer system. As we've seen, countries on the Bismarck Model generally have several, or many, different insurance plans. Germany has more than two hundred; Japan has more than two thousand. Canada has a separate government-run insurance fund for each of its provinces and territories. But these multipayer systems still provide the fairness and administrative simplicity of a single-payer structure; because all patients are treated the same, all the payers follow a coordinated set of rules and forms, and all providers' fees must adhere to a unified payment schedule.

A unified system makes it much easier to use digital record-keeping and smart cards like the *carte vitale* in France and the *Gesundheitskarte* in Germany. These digital records cut administrative costs, and they make for better medical care as well, because the doctor or pharmacist can instantly see what other treatment, tests, and medications the patient has received. The United States certainly has the technological skill to introduce digital medical records—in fact, that system I admired so much in France was designed in the USA. But we don't have a common record-keeping system here, because each of our overlapping systems and insurance companies has its own regimen.

Beyond that, a unified system eliminates the gamesmanship and cost-shifting that permeates American health care. In the United States, whichever entity is asked to pay for the treatment of a particular patient will save money if it can shove that patient off to another system. And so hospital emergency rooms try to push sick veterans out the door; why should the hospital pay for somebody's care when there's a separate VA health care system that could bear that cost? Some financial advisers counsel sick people on ways to *reduce* their net worth, so their medical bills can be shifted to Medicaid. If hospitals are underpaid by one payer—for example, Medicare—they make up the difference by raising their fees for other payers—for example, private insurance plans. In contrast, if there's only one system paying for care, there's no need to shuffle patients around and play paperwork games to shift the cost.

Beyond that, a single system for all creates an incentive for preventive health measures. As we've seen, U.S. insurance companies generally don't want to pay for preventive medicine, because the customer will likely have switched to another company or another system (like Medicare) long before there is any payoff for the investment in preventive care. In contrast, a system that covers everybody for the full extent of their lives will probably find it pays off to spend some money early in a patient's life to keep him healthy when he's older.

In every country (except, perhaps, a police state like Cuba), there is one group of citizens who are not bound by the unified health care system: the rich. Rich people everywhere have the wherewithal to get whatever medical treatment they want, when they want it, regardless of what the national system might provide. If all else fails, they just get on a jet to Rochester, Minnesota, and drop by the Mayo Clinic. In most countries, rich people are still required to pay the insurance premium, or the health care tax, that everybody else has to pay. But if they have enough money to buy care outside of the system, it's hard to stop them. Germany permits the richest 10 percent of the population to opt out of the health insurance system entirely; the Germans have concluded that rich people will get care one way or another, and getting that group out of the normal system relieves pressure on the sickness funds. (But it's not much relief. Many of the Germans who are entitled to opt out stick with the insurance system anyway, on grounds that it is cheaper and easier than buying medicine privately.) Similarly, people can buy private insurance in Britain and use it to pay the bills for those famous Harley Street doctors who operate outside the National Health Service. But most people choose the national system; only about 3 percent of Britain's medical costs are paid by private insurance.

In some societies—those with the most egalitarian traditions—the notion that a millionaire might jump the queue, or have access to a new experimental drug that the average man can't get, is offensive. Consequently, some countries (e.g., Sweden, Canada) have tried to make it illegal to purchase health care outside of the system. Generally, these prohibitions don't work; in Canada, as we saw in chapter 8, the Supreme Court ruled that this kind of restriction violates the basic right of Canadians to buy what they want with their own money. This experience suggests what might happen in the United States if we moved toward a coordinated health care system that covered everybody: Rich Americans would have to pay the same taxes or mandated insurance premiums as everybody else, but they would be able to buy care outside the system. A whole pocket industry would spring up to serve these upper-bracket customers who don't want to take part in the common system. If that happened, the health care system would look like the public school system: Everybody has to pay to support the public schools, and all have equal access to them. But people who want to use their own money for a private school are free to do so. That's the pattern with health care in all the other developed countries.

It may be possible to provide fair and cost-efficient health care for all while maintaining separate systems for the elderly, for the poor, for veterans, for renal-failure patients, for military personnel, for Native Americans, for working people, for members of Congress, and so on. It may be possible, but no country has ever made it work. That fragmented approach to health care clearly hasn't worked in the United States, which pays more and gets less in return than the rest of the industrialized world. And no other developed country wants to try it.

NONPROFIT FINANCING

Another basic building block in the health care systems of every wealthy country—except the United States—is the principle that financing health care must be a nonprofit endeavor. There's a crucial distinction between providing health care—what doctors, hospitals, labs, and pharmacies do—and financing health care. As we've seen around the world, most countries rely on free-market enterprise to provide health care—but not to pay for it. In the Beveridge Model nations and the National Health Insurance nations, health care finance is left to the government, through a mandatory national insurance scheme funded through general taxes, or through a dedicated tax just for health insurance. In the Bismarck Model, medical bills are paid by private but nonprofit insurance plans. In most countries an insurance company or sickness fund that runs a surplus at the end of the year has to redistribute that profit to the funds that lost money during that year.

The fundamental difference here is that foreign health insurance plans exist only to pay people's medical bills, not to make a profit. The United States is the only nation that lets insurance companies extract a profit from basic health coverage. This is the explanation for Myth 4 above: Health insurance companies don't have to be cruel to their customers if they don't have to worry about paying dividends to investors. But insurance firms whose primary mission is to make a profit quickly realize that covering every applicant and paying every claim will eat into profits. So they deny coverage to those who need it most, reject claims by the bucketful, and search for ways to rescind coverage just when the big bills roll in. That's why U.S. health insurance companies are loathed by their customers but loved on Wall Street. That's why health care economists around the world say that there's a basic conflict between the principle of health insurance and the pursuit of profit.

In the Bismarck Model countries, this principle is reflected in the rules governing health insurance. In those countries, everybody has to buy the basic package of health insurance—even the young and healthy, who may feel they don't need any coverage. This requirement, known to economists as the "individual mandate," has become intensely controversial in the United States. The 2010 health reform act includes a mild version of the individual mandate. But that portion of the law has been challenged in the courts by many states. So the "individual mandate" remains an unsettled issue for the United States. But in the rest of the world, there's no debate on this point. Everybody is mandated to pay into the insurance system; that guarantees enough income so that the plans can pay all the claims. The insurance plans, in turn, are required to accept all applicants, to pay all claims, and to continue coverage even when the insured gets hit by a truck and runs up large medical expenses. They can't make a profit on basic coverage, although insurance companies in many countries are permitted to sell for-profit policies covering services not included in the standard package of benefits.

It may be possible to finance fair and cost-efficient health care for all through profit-making health insurance. It may be possible, but no country has ever made it work. For-profit health insurance clearly hasn't worked in the United States, which spends more than any other country and still leaves millions without any coverage. And no other developed country wants to try it.

UNIVERSAL COVERAGE

As we've seen throughout this book, every developed country except the United States has designed a health care system that covers every resident. That's why St. Mary's Hospital in London gave my daughter immediate and competent care for her swollen ear, for free, less than a week after we arrived in Britain. These countries give everybody access to a doctor partly as a moral issue. But health officials in all the countries I visited told me that universal coverage also has pragmatic benefits that make any health care system cheaper and more effective.

This realization helps us answer the question: Which problem should America tackle first? The various shortcomings of the U.S. health care system can be summarized in three words: cost, coverage, and quality. When we set out to fix our system, where should we start? At first blush, it might seem logical to go after health care costs first; once costs are under control, we could more easily afford universal coverage. But everywhere I went on my global quest, I was told that this approach gets things backward. Universal coverage has to come first. Universal coverage is an essential tool to control costs and maintain the overall quality of a nation's health.

Covering everybody in a unified system creates a powerful political dynamic for managing the cost of health care. Since the costs of medical care are rising around the world, every health care system has to find ways to limit expenses—either by limiting the procedures and medications it will pay for, or by cutting the price it pays for the procedures that are covered. If everybody is covered, then everybody has an interest in seeing costs controlled; after all, if the system pays too much for my neighbor's Botox treatment, it may not have enough money to treat my broken shoulder. In a democracy, universal coverage helps create the political will to accept limitations and cost-control measures within the system. In any country, any decision to ration medical care is going to be unpopular with somebody. But if everyone is included in the health care system, people are more likely to accept a necessary but unpopular decision, because it leaves more money to treat everybody else.

Universal coverage also enhances health care results by improving the overall health of a nation. If everyone has access to a doctor, then people can get the diagnostic and preventive treatment that will keep them healthy. One of the major reasons the United States ranks low, compared to other rich nations, in standard measures of health care quality is that millions of Americans don't get any care until they are acutely ill. Universal access to diagnostic and preventive care also reduces costs, because it is much cheaper to treat a problem early than to take heroic medical measures when the illness becomes life-threatening.

It may be possible to provide fair and effective health care for everybody in a system where tens of millions of people have no insurance coverage. It may be possible, but no country has ever made it work. In the United States, our incomplete coverage is a key reason that twenty-two thousand of our fellow citizens die every year from diseases that could have been treated if they'd had health insurance. No other developed country wants to do things the way we do.

BEYOND THOSE PRACTICAL REASONS for universal coverage, of course, there's the basic moral imperative. Does a wealthy country have an ethical obligation to provide access to health care for everybody? Do we want to live in a society that lets tens of thousands of our neighbors die each year, and hundreds of thousands face financial ruin, because they can't afford medical care when they're sick? This, of course, is the "first question" that Professor William Hsiao asks whenever he reviews a country's health care system. And on this question, too, every developed country except the United States has reached the same conclusion: Everybody should have access to medical care. Having made that decision, the other nations have organized health care systems to meet that fundamental moral goal. If the United States made the same moral choice to provide universal coverage, then we, too could design a fair, efficient, and high-quality health care system for all Americans. And the principles we've learned from studying the other industrialized democracies will help us create that new health care system.

At the start of the twenty-first century, the world's richest and most powerful nation does not have the world's best health care system. But we could. Given our country's remarkable medical assets—the best-educated doctors and nurses, the most advanced facilities, the most innovative research research on earth, a strong infrastructure of preventive medicine—the United States could be, and should be, providing its citizens the finest health care in the world. We can heal America's ailing health care system—and the world's other industrialized democracies can show us how to do it.

AN AFTERWORD

"Obamacare" Explained

THE REFORM BILL THAT PRESIDENT BARACK OBAMA SIGNED into law on March 23, 2010—known formally as Public Law 111-148: The Patient Protection and Affordable Care Act,[1] and informally as "Obamacare"—is the most consequential and far-reaching health care law to emerge from Congress since the creation of Medicare and Medicaid in 1965.

If it works as planned, this multifaceted legislation will substantially expand health insurance coverage in the United States; it will outlaw many of the mechanisms American health insurers have used to avoid paying people's doctor bills; it will impose billions in new taxes, mainly on the rich; it will increase the pay of primary care doctors; it will make McDonald's, Dairy Queen, etc. provide the calorie count for every shake and burger; it might slow the relentless growth of U.S. medical costs.

And yet, it's important to recognize what the new law will not do. It does not simplify the crazy quilt of conflicting and overlapping payment systems that adds hundreds of billions of dollars each year to our national medical bill. It does not get us to universal coverage, a goal all the other industrialized democracies achieved long ago.

The reform package is so long (406,887 words, about four times the length of this book) and so broad (among much else, it restructures the U.S. student loan program) that most members of Congress didn't know precisely what was in it when they voted for or against the bill. Shortly after the first version of the legislation passed both houses of Congress, I got to attend a policy briefing for the members. As an economist checked off the countless new programs, prohibitions, authorizations, initiatives, and taxes in the bill, I noticed that the Senators and Representatives were all diligently taking notes about the bill they had just approved.

To understand this intricate legislative contraption, it helps to group the provisions of the law into four categories: (1) Expanded coverage; (2) Insurance regulation; (3) Taxes and other funding; (4) All the other stuff.

1. EXPANDED COVERAGE: The number of Americans without health insurance has been increasing steadily for decades, reaching nearly 50 million in 2010. The new law will reverse that trend and provide coverage to millions of people who can't get it today. How many millions is not clear, but the Congressional Budget Office estimates that as many as 32 million more people could have some form of health insurance by the year 2019. (That's the good news; the bad news is that the same office predicts about 23 million Americans will still be uninsured in 2019.)

   This expansion of coverage occurs in two major ways: Medicaid and private insurance.[2]

   Half of the increase will come from easing the qualifications for Medicaid, the government program that provides free or subsidized health care for low-income families. By

expanding the definition of "low-income," and by including
those without children, the law should allow about 16 million
additional uninsured people to get medical treatment under
Medicaid. The late Nikki White, the thirty-two-year-old
lupus victim we met on the first page of this book, would
likely have qualified for Medicaid under the new rules—
and would have had a good chance to live. Normally, the cost
of Medicaid is split between the federal government and each
state; under the new law, Washington will pay all the costs of
the expanded coverage for the first five years. Obama says that
he "hopes" the states will support the Medicaid expansion
after this supplemental federal funding ends.

Through the new law, another large group—perhaps as
many as 16 million uninsured Americans—will get access to
private health insurance plans that they can't get, or can't afford, now. As of 2014, each state will have to set up an insurance "exchange." Essentially, that means an online market,
like the Web sites that sell books or airline tickets. People who
don't get insurance through their employer can go to this mar-
ketplace and find a choice of plans from various insurance
companies. The law says that each exchange should offer
five different levels of coverage plans ("Bronze," "Silver,"
"Gold," "Platinum," and "Catastrophic") to give buyers a
broad choice.

Because nobody knows how much insurance premiums
will cost in 2014, the law includes federal tax credits to help
families pay for this insurance. And the program is generous;
families with income as high as $88,000 per year can get
some of this subsidy.

The law requires all employers with more than forty-nine
people on the payroll to provide a health insurance plan for
employers. It offers a tax credit for smaller companies that

provide health insurance. The mandate on bigger companies doesn't kick in until 2014, but the tax credit for small employers began in 2010. This timing reflected the Democrats' fervent desire to provide concrete benefits of the reform plan before the 2010 Congressional elections, but to delay the costs of the plan until well after.

One much-discussed idea that did not get into the final version of the bill was a so-called public option—that is, a nonprofit health insurance plan offered by the federal government, a sort of Medicare-at-any-age program. Fearful of competition from the government, the health insurance industry lobbied strenuously, and successfully, to kill the public option plan. But the mere threat of a government-run competitor had a profound effect: to ward off the public option, the insurers reluctantly agreed to a broad range of new restrictions and regulations that they had never accepted before.

2. INSURANCE REGULATION: The 2010 law bans, for the first time, several of the crueler practices that private health insurers have used over the years to avoid paying their customers' bills—and thus enhance their profits. Because this was probably the most popular aspect of the reform plan, President Obama almost always referred to his proposal not as "health care reform," but rather as "health insurance reform." With these changes, the American health insurance companies will be more like—but still not just like—the insurers we have seen in other Bismarck-model countries.

The most important new rule is called "guaranteed issue." Beginning in 2014, insurers will be required to issue, or renew, a policy to anybody, regardless of any preexisting condition. This change alone should provide coverage to some 20 million Americans who cannot get coverage now. (Until this rule takes effect in 2014, states are supposed to expand their existing "high-risk" insurance programs so that more of these uninsurables can be covered.)

As we've seen throughout this book, though, the principle of "guaranteed issue" can only work if it is coupled with another rule, the "individual mandate"—that is, the requirement that everybody buy insurance. The insurers need the mandated customer base to have a broad enough risk pool to pay for guaranteed issue. All the other rich countries figured out this connection long ago; the 2010 act marks the first time the United States has coupled these two requirements.

But there's a problem in the reform law: The individual mandate is not firmly established. Congress flinched at the idea of setting a strict penalty for people who don't buy insurance; the result will likely be that many healthy people will choose to dodge the mandate.

Beyond that, some prominent conservatives have filed a lawsuit saying the individual mandate is unconstitutional. The legal theory here has a purist libertarian appeal: How dare Big Government dictate that I buy a particular product? Unfortunately for the libertarians, that argument has been settled in the United States for two centuries. There are all sorts of government mandates to buy things. It's illegal to walk down the street naked in any American city. That's a mandate to buy clothes. People are jailed for failing to feed their children; that's a government mandate to buy food.

The fate of the individual mandate provision is pivotal. If it fails, then guaranteed issue will fail as well. And that would pretty much cut the heart out of the Patient Protection and Affordable Care Act.

Beyond that basic requirement, the reform law outlaws the reprehensible insurance practice of "rescission," where the company accepts your premium payment every month as long as you're healthy, but then rescinds, or cancels, your coverage when you face big medical bills. The law prohibits insurers from setting annual or lifetime limits on reimbursement, so that people don't find their coverage terminated while still in the hospital. And the law requires insurers to keep their administrative costs down to 20 percent of premium income for most plans. That's a significant change. But it means the U.S. insurers can still have paperwork costs four times as high as the German, French, Swiss, and Japanese health insurance companies we've seen in this book.

Even with the new restrictions, American health insurance companies will get away with some practices that are banned in every other rich democracy. The U.S. firms will still be allowed to deny your claims (although they will have to report, for the first time, how many claims they reject each year). When they do pay, they can still take weeks or months to do so, without the strict time limits that are common elsewhere. And the United States will continue to be the only developed nation that permits health insurance companies to make a profit on the basic package of coverage.

3. TAXES AND OTHER FUNDING: The "Obamacare" package of legislation is projected to cost at least $940 billion over the first ten years.[3] To raise that money, Congress imposed new taxes and fees on some of the industries that have been big winners under the current health care system. Drug companies, medical device makers, and health insurance companies will all be hit with new taxes. There's also a new federal sales tax on tanning salons, justified on the theory that tanning can cause skin cancer, so the salons increase the national health care bill.

Beginning in 2013, the bill also raises the Medicare tax for people earning more than $200,000 per year (or couples earning over \$250,000). For those wealthy earners, the tax to pay for Medicare will jump from 2.9 percent to 3.8 percent. The most striking change in tax policy is that the same 3.8 percent Medicare tax will also be applied, for the first time, to financial earnings for people in those upper brackets. Formerly, workers who earned a paycheck had to pay Social Security and Medicare taxes, but those who got their income from finance—interest, dividends, capital gains, etc.—were exempt. Under the new law, rich investors, too, will help pay for Medicare.

The law also imposes penalty fees on individuals who don't buy health insurance—that's the impact of the individual mandate—and on large employers that don't help their workers buy health insurance. There's also a new tax on the most generous health insurance plans; that one will be felt by top-tier executives, but also by hourly workers whose unions have negotiated lavish health coverage.

The bill cuts some taxpayer subsidies paid to insurance companies that operate so-called Medicare Advantage plans. Like almost all major federal initiatives, the reform plan also maintains that large sums can be saved by eliminating waste and fraud.

4. ALL THE OTHER STUFF: The law will provide subsidies for seniors who can't afford to pay for their prescriptions under Medicare. It requires chain restaurants and vending machines to list the calorie count for everything they sell. It creates a new federal program to pay (\$50 per day) for long-term care; this starts small, but could grow into a major new entitlement program. To induce more medical students into family practice, the law will help pay the medical school debt of primary care doctors and sharply raises Medicaid payments for primary care. The plan sets up a new federal agency, the

Independent Payment Advisory Board, to recommend how much Medicare should pay doctors and hospitals for each medical procedure. With the right leadership, this board could impose the kind of cost controls that we saw at work in France, Japan, and elsewhere and thus reduce the constant growth in American health care costs.

In sum, the Patient Protection and Affordable Care Act—it's already known in Washington by the acronym PPACA, pronounced "pea-packah"—should extend insurance coverage to millions of Americans who are uninsured now and end some of the insurance companies' harsher practices. But the sad truth is that, even with this ambitious reform, the United States will still have the most complicated, the most expensive, and the most inequitable health care system of any developed nation. The new law won't get us to the destination all the other industrialized democracies have reached: universal health care coverage at reasonable cost. To achieve that goal, the United States will still have to take some lessons from the other national health care systems described in this book.

Appendix: The Best Health Care System in the World

In the beginning, I thought the quest for a cure for our nation's health care problems would be fairly easy. I'd find a country that had a longer life expectancy than the United States has. I'd find a country with better cost control in its medical system. I'd find a system with fairer access to health care. Then I'd figure out which nation offered the best combination of those three measures. Voilà! I'd have the model we could transplant into the American health care system. And in the process, I figured, I'd probably find a country with great doctors who could do something about my aching shoulder.

In fact, the process turned out to be more complicated than that. For one thing, as we've seen, every industrialized country has fairer access to health care and lower costs for health care than the United States, so those conditions didn't narrow down the search at all. Most of the world's wealthy countries have longer life expectancies than we do, too. According to the CIA data for 2006, five small, wealthy enclaves—Andorra, Macau, Singapore, San Marino, and Hong Kong—lead the world in longevity, with all five reporting that an average child born in 2006 was expected to live about eighty-two years. Among the major nations, Japan has the longest life expectancy at birth, with a combined male-female average of 81.25 years. Switzerland, Sweden, Australia, and Canada also have a life expectancy of eight decades. The saddest countries on this score are poor African nations plagued by AIDS and civil unrest: countries such as Zimbabwe (39 years), Angola (38), Lesotho (34), Botswana (33.7), and, finally, Swaziland, a troubled, land-locked southeast African nation of 712,000 people, where the average baby born in 2006 could expect to die at the age of 32 years and seven months.[1]

On this measure—average life expectancy at birth—the United States comes in at 77.85 years. That means the world's richest country ranks forty-seventh, just ahead of Cyprus and a little behind Bosnia and Herzegovina, in terms of longevity. The United States is among the worst of the industrialized nations on this score; for that matter, the average American can expect a shorter life than people in relatively poor countries like Jordan. Experts offer several reasons for our country's low ranking; among other things, the World Health Organization says, America's unusually high rate of homicide is one reason we die younger than the Japanese, the Canadians, or the Greeks.[2] But the quality of, and access to, national health care plays a large role in any country's average life expectancy; the fact that tens of millions of us don't have access to a doctor means Americans are dying of health problems that would probably be cured in any other developed country.

The bigger issue, though, is that life expectancy by itself isn't a very useful measure of anything. The experts who study vital statistics and health systems all agree that expected longevity at birth is a crude test at best of a nation's health status. Consider a woman who is ninety-two years old, bedridden with assorted diseases. She's unable to get up, dress herself, or tie her shoes; she doesn't recognize her children; she often feels pain on waking, in which case she is given drugs that relieve the distress but leave her in a state of oblivion. At some cost, modern medicine can extend her life span to, perhaps, ninety-seven years—and we often do. In many nations, including ours, doctors and nurses would generally be required by law to keep her alive as long as medical science makes it possible. Multiplied a few thousand times, that kind of treatment will increase a nation's average life expectancy. But how much good was achieved, for the patient, for her family, for society as a whole? What does the number of bedridden ninety-five-year-olds tell us about the quality of a nation's health care?

Questions like that are largely the province of a relatively new academic discipline, health care economics. This field was started in the 1960s by the American Nobel laureate Kenneth Arrow. As with many other areas of contemporary economics, most of its leading lights are Americans—not surprising, given that health care spending now represents about one-sixth of the entire American economy. The analytic studies and the mathematical models of the health care economists are essential to the design of effective health care systems; they were extremely helpful to me during my global medical odyssey.

To CARRY OUT comparative studies of different health care systems, the health care economists have come up with a range of measures of a nation's health status that are more sophisticated and more meaningful than "life expectancy at birth." One important gauge is the DALE, or Disability-Adjusted Life Expectancy, an index developed by economists and statisticians at the World Health Organization. (Sometimes this same concept is given a slightly different name, the HALE, for Health-Adjusted Life Expectancy.) A nation's DALE rating—sometimes described by the term "healthy life expectancy"—measures how many years the average citizen can expect to live before encountering the disabling diseases of old age. The basic theory is that most people live in a state of "full health." In this condition, you feel good most of the time. You may have an illness or accident now and then, but a healthy person recovers from it. At some point, though, "full health" gives way to illness. The chronic diseases we generally associate with the elderly begin to take a toll: heart disease, back pain, rheumatoid arthritis, blindness, hearing loss, Alzheimer's, and so on. At that point, people are living in "partial health." Some people with these problems can go on living with only minor impairment of their normal activities. Others may be so sick or disabled that their life isn't close to what they enjoyed in the years of "full health." The World Health Organization developed a complicated set of formulas to weight these ailments according to the level of severity. A person living with a painful cancer, for example, might be rated at one-fourth as healthy as a person in "full health." Then each additional year that this cancer patient lives would be rated at one-fourth of a year on the Disability-Adjusted Life Expectancy scale. The WHO found that, on average, a country's "healthy life expectancy" is about seven years shorter than the straightforward "life expectancy at birth." A high ranking on the DALE score means that a nation's population has good health habits and that the country provides good access to medical care, for both prevention and cure of disease.[3]

On the DALE measure, the country with the longest healthy life expectancy is Japan, where the average baby born today can expect to live 74.5 years in "full health." The top ten countries for healthy living, in terms of DALE years, are:

1.	Japan	74.5 years
2.	Australia	73.2 years
3.	France	73.1 years
4.	Sweden	73.0 years
5.	Spain	72.8 years

(continued)

6. Italy	72.7 years
7. Greece	72.5 years
8. Switzerland	72.5 years
9. Monaco	72.4 years
10. Andorra	72.3 years

Source: World Health Organization, The World Health Report 2000.

According to the World Health Organization, twenty-four countries have a healthy life expectancy of 70 years or more; about one hundred countries have a DALE between 60 and 70. Once again, the ten saddest countries in the world were sub-Saharan African nations beset by AIDS, poverty, and civil strife. Sierra Leone, a nation of 4.3 million on Africa's Atlantic coast, came up last on this ranking; a baby born there today can expect to live in "full health" for less than 26 years.

The richest country in the world ranked twenty-fourth in the world for healthy life expectancy, with a DALE of 70 years (72.6 years for females and 67.5 years for males). That put the United States just behind Israel and just ahead of Cyprus. Again, we stand below almost all the other developed nations. "The position of the United States is one of the major surprises of the ranking system," noted Christopher Murray, a doctor and health economist at Harvard who helped design the DALE formula. "Basically, you die earlier and spend more time disabled if you're an American rather than a member of most other advanced countries." Still, the U.S. ranking in DALE terms, twenty-fourth, is considerably higher than the forty-seventh place we scored on the simpler ranking of life expectancy at birth. That difference means that American health care is making people healthier—at least, for those who have access to it. It's because we fail to provide access to regular health care for 45 million Americans that our overall rank for healthy life expectancy trails the rest of the developed world.

The basic concept of the DALE is "disability adjustment," the notion that the years of a person's life should be classified as periods of "full health" and various degrees of "partial health." Once you get used to this idea, you can start to grasp two other key concepts that health planners rely on: the QALY (pronounced "quolly") and the DALY ("dolly"). These two important measures—the quality-adjusted life year (QALY) and the disability-adjusted life year (DALY)—are used by health care planners around the world to set priorities. They help decide which medical treatments or drugs are worth spending money on, and which ones don't provide a significant return for the money spent.[4]

Suppose, for example, that you're the health minister of a country called Saludia, and you have to allocate the money in your national budget for health care among various problems. Naturally, different people have different ideas about how that money should be spent. The children of elderly people with Alzheimer's disease are clamoring for $50 million in additional spending for assisted-living facilities where their suffering parents can get the daily help they need to stay alive. The association of cardiac surgeons is calling for $50 million extra to fund operations implanting coated stents in the arteries of cardiovascular patients. Meanwhile, the national union of psychiatrists and their patients are demanding $50 million more in the health budget to pay for drugs that control depression. At the same time, the national office of public health is asking for $50 million to finance a campaign to stop people from smoking. As the health minister, how do you decide which of these investments would be the most useful in increasing overall national health? Which one would provide the most extra years of healthy life for the people of Saludia?

To answer that question, a health minister looks at the QALYs. This concept measures both the number of years of life gained by a particular operation or drug or informational campaign, and the quality of the years gained. Continued treatment of a bedridden Alzheimer's patient might provide five more calendar years of life but not five QALYs. In contrast, spending the same amount of money to help a young mother control her depression would improve the quality of life both for the mother and for her children and thus purchase many more QALYs than an equal investment in treating the elderly.

Measuring QALYs is both easy and difficult, because it involves counting years and judging "quality." The counting part is simple: Somebody lives ninety-two years or ninety-seven. But the measure of health quality quickly becomes touchy. Economists have devised a descending scale of "health states" ranging from one to zero. If you have no mental or physical health problems, if you are living a normal, active life without pain or impairment, then your health state is rated at 1.0. If you're dead, your health state is rated zero. There are all sorts of gradations in between.

If you're basically healthy, not anxious or depressed, but have "some problems with performing usual activities, some pain or discomfort," then your health state is rated at 0.76. (That probably describes me and my bad shoulder.) If you are moderately anxious or depressed, "unable to wash or dress self, unable to perform usual activities, with moderate pain or discomfort," your health state falls to 0.079. And some people have a health state that is scored below zero—that is, worse than dead. A patient who is "confined to bed; unable to wash or dress self; unable to perform usual activities; in extreme pain or discomfort; moderately anxious or depressed" would be rated at a "health state" of −0.429.[5] To put this number into plain English, the economists rate that patient's health state as better off dead. But she and her grandchildren might prefer to see her stay alive a while longer.

If you embrace the concept of the QALY, then the delicate budget decisions facing the health minister of Saludia become somewhat easier to resolve. There are formulae to calculate the gains, in quality-adjusted life years, from different kinds of medical treatments and campaigns. Paying for assisted living for a bedridden patient who will gain virtually nothing in terms of "quality-adjusted" years is essentially throwing away money by this measure, since no QALYs will be gained. Paying for the implant of ventricular stents will keep some cardiac patients alive but at major cost; in the United States, the stent surgery would cost $900,000 for each QALY gained. By comparison, drugs that can control depression turn out to be a bargain, costing $20,000 per QALY (antidepression treatment doesn't necessarily extend the length of life but improves its quality). The most productive expenditure of all, in terms of gaining years of healthy life, would be to promote nonsmoking; that costs only $7,200 for each QALY gained.

What's really happening with DALEs/HALEs, DALYs, QALYs, and similar tests for allocating health care resources is that this economic mumbo jumbo is invoked to conceal difficult value judgments about life and death. Consider, for example, this common dilemma: There's a healthy kidney available for transplant and two patients with an acute need for it. How does a health system choose between the two potential recipients? What if one patient is wealthy and well-connected and the other a part-time janitor at Wal-Mart? Should that matter? What if one of the patients is a decorated Army veteran who fought for her country, and the other runs an Internet porn site? Should that matter? The QALY/DALY approach, focusing on the number of healthy years to be saved, would generally steer that lone kidney to the younger of the two patients (regardless of wealth, background, or occupation), on the theory that it will probably provide more healthy life years in a recipient who is fifty than in one who is eighty.

The same kind of value judgments are necessarily wrapped into any effort to rank national health care systems. Any measure of "quality of life" or "degree of disability" is bound to be subjective. A paraplegic who has adjusted well to life in a wheelchair might consider his quality of life to be fine, while a dedicated soccer player might look on the same legless life as unbearable. Once you start measuring "quality" and "disability," the measure of any country's national health status will require arbitrary definitions of those terms. If considerations such as "equity" in access to health care or "fairness" in the financing of health care are thrown into the ranking as well, even more value judgments are required. On top of that, any effort to rank the world's nations in some kind of league table is likely to run up against national pride; patriotic Americans (or Cubans or Chinese) who want to believe that "We're Number One" will not easily accept a ranking that says the United States (or Cuba or China) does not have the best health care system in the world.

That explains the frosty reception—in the United States, at least—that greeted the most ambitious effort ever made to grade the national health care systems of different countries.

At the start of the twenty-first century, the World Health Organization, a United Nations agency based in Geneva, produced an unprecedented work of analysis: a comprehensive and detailed study of health status and the health care systems in each of its 191 member nations. Four years in the making, the WHO's *World Health Report, 2000,* "Health Systems: Improving Performance," was designed to help the WHO's member nations improve their health care systems by studying "best practices" in the countries that provided the best care. "Improving the performance of health systems around the world is the *raison d'être* of this report," wrote the WHO's director-general, Gro Harlem Brundtland, an M.D. who had previously been the Prime Minister of Norway.[6]

Governments, think tanks, universities, and international organizations churn out ambitious studies like that all the time; a common result of such endeavors is that the thick summary report and the countless supporting documents are put up on a shelf somewhere to gather dust, essentially ignored for the rest of time. To avoid that ignominious fate, the people in charge of the WHO study hit on a strategy that was guaranteed to make their report a global phenomenon. In addition to the extensive analysis of the financing, the organization, and the operation of different countries' health care systems, the WHO team decided to rank all the world's national health care systems, from No. 1 to No. 191—to designate the best and the worst health care systems on earth and all the countries in between in order of overall performance.

This PR gambit worked beautifully. Editors, producers, and politicians found it impossible to ignore a serious study by a distinguished international body that delineated precisely where each country ranked vis-à-vis its neighbors, its allies, and its enemies. The Greeks (No. 14 overall) were delighted that they outranked their archrivals, the Turks (No. 70). The South Koreans (No. 58) trumpeted their huge victory over North Korea (No. 167). The wealthy oil state of Oman was thrilled with its No. 8 standing in the world, particularly because it ranked a full fourteen countries higher than the wealthy oil state of United Arab Emirates, right next door. Americans, in contrast, were not pleased to be told that their extravagant spending on health care produced results that ranked the United States thirty-seventh in the world—lower than Colombia, Costa Rica, Malta, and Morocco. No American wanted to march through the streets chanting "We're Number 37!" And thus, unlike so many other heavy-duty policy reports, "Health Systems: Improving Performance" drew front-page headlines and extensive commentary all over the world. It remains a staple of discussion and debate whenever health policy officials and scholars gather for international meetings.

The problem with this ingenious attention-getting strategy was that it was not simple to carry out. It was all but impossible to design a single rating scale that would accommodate countries ranging from Monaco (population, 33,000; per capita income, $30,000 per year) to Nigeria (population, 101 million; per capita income, $310 per year); from Japan, where the average person goes to the doctor fourteen times per year, to India, where hundreds of millions never see a doctor at all. The WHO research team, led by Dr. Christopher Murray of Harvard and Julio Frenk, the former health minister of Mexico, dealt with this concern by producing a number of different ranking systems, which are found scattered over ten separate "Annex Tables" at the end of the long report.

The simplest scale was the DALE rating: how long the average person in a given country could expect to live without serious illness or disability (or, as the WHO report describes it, "the expectation of life lived in equivalent full health"). As discussed earlier in this appendix, Japan led the world on that ranking and Sierra Leone ranked last. The United States came in at twenty-fourth, behind most of the other developed countries.

The WHO study also graded something it called "responsiveness" of national health care systems. This was a measure of how customer-friendly the national medical structure is: Does the doctor respect the patient's dignity? Does the system protect the privacy of personal medical information? Does a patient get prompt treatment or wait months to see a specialist? Does the patient have freedom to choose among doctors and hospitals? On this criterion, and this one alone, the United States rated No. 1 in the world, followed by the other wealthy democracies of western Europe, Japan, and Canada. The worst countries in terms of responsiveness to patients were the poor countries of Africa.

But the USA did not fare as well on two key issues that the WHO counted as more important than responsiveness. Those were "goodness" and "fairness." The "goodness" test measured how well a country did at keeping its people healthy—essentially, the DALE, or "healthy life expectancy" measure. The "fairness" test measured two things:

1. How equally a health system treated the rich and the poor.
2. How a national health care system was financed. For the WHO, a progressive financing system, in which rich people paid more than the poor to finance health care for all, was an essential element of "fairness."

The United States, with tens of millions of low-income people left out of its health insurance system and thus forced to pay out of pocket for whatever treatment they could get, came out badly on both measures of "fairness." In terms of equal distribution of health care, the United States was ranked thirty-second in the world. Chile, Japan, and the European democracies stood at the top of this table. In terms of "Fairness of financial contribution," the United States was rated fifty-fourth. Colombia, with health care funded by a steeply progressive tax code, topped the chart on this scale, followed closely by western European countries and Japan.

Finally, the WHO experts took all these factors, tabulated each country's score on each measure, and arrived at its rating of "overall performance." But this score was adjusted by one more fudge factor: a comparison of each country's actual performance on national health care to the overall performance it should have been able to achieve, considering its level of education and the amount of money it spends on health care. With this ultimate wrinkle factored in, the report finally came up with its ranking of "overall performance" in all 191 member nations. When the figures were all computed, the French health care system was rated first in the world—and the United States, thirty-seventh. The top ten health systems in this composite ranking were:

1. France
2. Italy
3. San Marino
4. Andorra
5. Malta
6. Singapore
7. Spain
8. Oman
9. Austria
10. Japan

Predictably, this widely reported WHO ranking drew loud hurrahs from the countries that ranked well, and angry criticism from those that came in lower than they expected. The critics argued that the whole idea of a single rating scale for 191 countries was questionable, and that the methodology the WHO used to develop its "overall performance" score for each country was so complicated that hardly anybody could figure it out. On the other hand, the WHO study did tend to confirm a general sense among health care officials and academics around the world about the best national health care systems. The major countries rating highly on the various WHO scorecards—Japan, France, Germany, Sweden—were already recognized by health officials around the world as exemplars of good overall health and of fair and effective health care.

One repeated point of criticism of "Health Systems: Improving Performance" was that all the assessments in the World Health Organization's global comparisons were done by experts—doctors, public health officials, economists, statisticians, and the like. The only people the WHO didn't bother to ask were the patients. There was no public input into the WHO study, no measure of how satisfied the people in each country were with the health care they received.

Accordingly, a research team at the Harvard School of Public Health launched a sort of counter-WHO comparison of health care systems in 2001, based not on expert opinion but, rather, on the perception of the patients, as reflected in national opinion surveys. (The Harvard study looked at fifteen European countries, the United States, and Canada. It did not include Japan, which ranked at or near No. 1 in most of the WHO rankings.) In this "Satisfaction Survey," the United States finished near the bottom among developed countries, ranking fourteenth out of the seventeenth countries listed. In terms of public satisfaction with the national health care system, Denmark rated the highest, with 91 percent of Danes saying they were either "very" or "fairly" satisfied. Next in order were Finland (81 percent), Austria (73 percent), the Netherlands (70 percent), Luxembourg (67 percent), and France (65 percent). Only 40 percent of Americans declared themselves satisfied with our health care system; Italy (20 percent), Portugal (16 percent), and Greece (16 percent) ranked even lower than the United States by this measure.[7]

The Commonwealth Fund, a private research organization based in New York, regularly carries out a different comparative study of health care systems: The "National Scorecard," designed primarily to gauge how well the United States stacks up against the world's other wealthy countries. The United States basically flunks this test, coming in at or near the bottom on most of the fund's measures of health care access and quality. "The United States is the only major industrialized country that fails to guarantee universal health insurance," the Scorecard concluded in 2006. "The U.S. Health System is not the best on quality of care, nor is it a leader in health information technology."[8] To measure the quality of health care in various countries, the Scorecard measured how many people in each country who contracted a potentially fatal but treatable medical condition were treated successfully and survived. Testing nineteen countries on this measure of "avoidable mortality," the Commonwealth Fund came up with this ranking of the world's best health systems:

---

1. France
2. Japan
3. Spain
4. Sweden
5. Italy
6. Australia
7. Canada
8. Norway

(continued)

9. Netherlands
10. Greece
11. Germany

. . .

15. United States

. . .

19. Portugal

THERE'S A FAIRLY DEPRESSING pattern for Americans in these international comparisons of health care systems. Generally, the same usual suspects come in near the top on every ranking, while the USA tends to get a mediocre grade every time. We do better than most of the world's poorer countries, but perform poorly compared to the other wealthy nations. And this fair-to-middling performance comes despite huge investment in health care. The area where the United States routinely leads every other country is in health care spending, both as per-capita expenditure and as a percentage of gross national product.

Still, there are experts who argue that American health care ranks with the best in the world. These advocates note that the United States has doctors, hospitals, research labs, and medical schools that lead the world when it comes to innovative high-tech approaches to acute and chronic medical problems. American medicine has more specialists, more technology, more groundbreaking experimentation than any other country, rich or poor. And the American reliance on private, for-profit health insurance companies for the bulk of medical coverage is in accord with American values of capitalism and freedom.

One of those defenders of American-style health care is Dr. Kevin C. Fleming, an internist at the Mayo Clinic in Minnesota and a health care analyst for the Heritage Foundation, a Washington think tank committed to free-market solutions to national problems. Dr. Fleming argues that "socialized medicine"—his term for the health care systems in other wealthy countries—doesn't match American medicine in quality of care. Here's a sample of his argument, focusing on medical care for newborns:

> There are many ways to measure quality. One way is to consider indices of treatment, such as neonatal care. Today, the United States has high neonatal intensive care capacity, with 6.1 neonatologists per 10,000 live births; Australia has 3.7 per 10,000; Canada has 3.3 per 10,000; and the United Kingdom, 2.7 per 10,000. The United States has 3.3 intensive care beds per 10,000 live births; Australia and Canada have 2.6 per 10,000; and the United Kingdom, 0.67 per 10,000. While American "overinvestment" in lifesaving of premature infants may come at the expense of proportionately less support for preconception and prenatal care, British neonatal intensive care capacity is far below that. . . . Although Canada has far more generous welfare entitlements, less income disparity, universal health coverage, and more uniform standards of perinatal care than the United States, variations in mortality rates among Canadian neonatal intensive care units appear to be as wide as those reported in the United States and elsewhere.[9]

Dr. Fleming's approach to the question reflects the general tenor of those who still say that the United States has "the best health care in the world." In economic terms, he deals mainly with "inputs." When it comes to numbers of specialists, numbers of beds, investment in intensive care facilities, the United States ranks near the top every time. But the discerning reader of this book may notice one statistic that Dr. Fleming did not mention in his comparative discussion of "indices of treatment" for newborns: What are the "outputs"? How does the United States perform, relative to other wealthy countries, when it comes to keeping sick babies alive? On this scorecard, as on so many others, the United States stands behind other developed nations. Here's a ranking of the infant mortality rate—a measure of the number of babies, per 1,000 births, who die before their first birthday—for several wealthy countries, using statistics from 2005:

INFANT MORTALITY RATES, 2008

Country	Deaths per 1,000 births
Sweden	2.76
Japan	2.8
Norway	3.64
France	3.41
Germany	4.08
Switzerland	4.2
Canada	4.63
UK	5.01
Cuba	6.04
United States	6.37

Source: CIA, World Factbook, 2009.

In summary, then, it is not as easy as it might seem to find "the best health care system in the world." Different studies produce different rankings; countries that excel in some areas do less well in others. Still, there is a coterie of developed countries that are providing quality health care, distributing it fairly and equitably—and doing all that for much less money than the United States is spending.

A Note of Thanks

Shortly after I launched into this book, I taught a one-semester course at Princeton University. While I was on campus, I wandered over to the Woodrow Wilson School of Public and International Affairs to sit in on a graduate seminar titled "WWS 597: The Political Economy of Health Systems." The syllabus was formidable, and much of the subject matter looked to be as dry as dust. But two minutes into the professor's first lecture, I realized that WWS 597 was going to be a great educational experience. That's because the professor was Uwe Reinhardt, a global leader in the field of health care economics—and a superb teacher. Professor Reinhardt seemed to know all the strengths and all the weaknesses of every health care system in the world. He imparted this information with wit and intensity and a passion for the subject that my fellow students and I found irresistible. In just about every seminar, Reinhardt recited the central point of his course, which has now become a central message of this book: "Every nation's health care system reflects that nation's basic moral values," he taught us. "Once a nation decides that it has a moral obligation to provide health care for everybody, then it can build a system to meet that obligation."

Uwe Reinhardt's instruction has informed every chapter of this book. Beyond that, Uwe also introduced me to other health care economists around the world. The academic experts have been generous with their time and their insights; their help has been a pearl of great price for a neophyte author taking on this imposing topic. I owe particular thanks to Tsung-Mei Cheng, the author of the Universal Laws of Health Care Systems cited in this book, and a key architect of Taiwan's system of universal health care. (Dr. Cheng also happens to be Mrs. Uwe Reinhardt.) Professor William Hsiao of Harvard showed me the basic building blocks of health care systems, the elements he used as he supervised the design and construction of systems for Taiwan and a dozen other countries. I received valuable help as well from Professor Ikegami Naoki, Professor Karl Lauterbach, Professor François Bonnaud, Nigel Hawkes, Cathy Schoen, and Drew Altman. These experts don't always agree with one another, and they don't always agree with me. So any errors in these pages are my fault, not theirs.

I am deeply grateful to the physicians around the world who took me in and gave me professional advice, both on health care systems and on sore shoulders. This generous group of healers includes Drs. Ahmed Badat and John Reidy in the UK; Drs. Bertrand Tamalet, François Bonnaud, and Hélène Bonnaud in France; Dr. Christina von Köckritz and her *Arzthelferin,* Antje Krickow, in Germany; Drs. Nakamichi Noriaki, Kono Keiko, and Kono Hitoshi in Japan; Drs. Chiu Wen-Ta and Li Mei-Li in Taiwan; Dr. Charles Favrod-Coune in Switzerland; Drs. Steve Goluboff and Noel Doig in Canada; and Dr. Sherab Tenzin in Nepal. I owe special thanks, both as a writer and as a patient, to my kind and skillful orthopedic surgeon, Dr. Donald Ferlic of Denver, Colorado, USA.

I relied heavily on the help of expert researchers around the world. I owe a particular debt to Allison Shepherd, Habibou Bangre, Beatrice

Shaad-Noble, Tania Shink, and Kate McMahon. Two veteran reporters of immeasurable skill, Adi Bloom in London and Togo Shigehiko in Tokyo, once again gave me priceless assistance. Sir Mark Tully shared his vast knowledge of India and Ayurveda.

My fellow travelers for the films based on this book played a large role in shaping the right questions for me to investigate in each country and helping me understand the answers. The companionship of Mark Rublee, Jon Palfreman, Steve Atlas, and Alex Palfreman significantly enhanced the pleasure of our far-flung days as we rode the bullet train past Mount Fuji, walked the Westminster Bridge beneath Big Ben, strolled the shore of Lake Geneva, braved the rickshaw route through Delhi's Chandni Chowk, rode bikes through the Brandenburg Gate, and dined on grilled snake in Taipei's Snake Alley.

Several friends and health care experts helped along the way by reading chunks of the manuscript. I'm particularly indebted to Richard Morgan, Tom Benghauser, Joe and Lynne Ptacek, and Wendy Liu, a student of mine who became my teacher as the work progressed. I'm grateful for access to the collections in the libraries of Princeton University, Keio University, the University of Denver, the University of Colorado Medical School, the Denver Public Library, and the Westminster Libraries in London. Dean Richard Krugman and Dr. Joel Levine of the University of Colorado Medical School kindly and patiently answered my health care questions.

The Kaiser Family Foundation (KFF) made me a Kaiser Media Fellow, providing not only research funds but cachet and entrée to the health care fraternity, which proved extremely helpful on my global travels. I can't say thank you often enough to Penny Duckham, Deirdre Graham, and Drew Altman of KFF for their kindness. I'm grateful to the Colorado Trust, the Colorado Health Foundation, and the Commonwealth Fund; those organizations, all dedicated to improving American health care, helped us make the films based on this book.

As she has done for me in the past, the great editor Ann Godoff dug through the manuscript of this book, found its real meaning, and figured out how to bring it to the fore. Lindsay Whalen of The Penguin Press displayed her characteristic intelligence, efficiency, and tact as she steered the book to publication. I'm grateful to Candy Gianetti for meticulous copyediting. My friend and agent, Gail Ross, once again realized the outline of my book before I did and kept me going through the tough times.

Last but foremost, Margaret Mary McMahon, McMahon Thomas Homer Reid, O'Gorman Catherine Penelope Reid, and Erin Margaret Andromache Wilhelmina Reid put up with the author and the manuscript in cheery fashion for years, a task much tougher than writing any book.

Denver, 2009

Notes

CHAPTER 1: A QUEST FOR TWO CURES

1. World Health Organization (hereafter WHO), *The World Health Report, 2000*, Annex Table 10, p. 200. As we'll see in the appendix, this study sparked intense controversy.
2. Robert Blendon et al., "The Public Versus the World Health Organization," *Health Affairs*, May/June 2001, p. 18.
3. Thomas Bodenheimer and Kevin Grumbach, *Understanding Health Policy: A Clinical Approach* (Lange Medical Books, 2005), 3.
4. For example, Heritage Foundation, *Backgrounder No. 1973*, September 22, 2006. This briefing paper reviews ideas for universal health coverage in the United States. The first sentence: "There is renewed interest in socialized medicine."
5. Dwight D. Eisenhower, *At Ease* (Fort Washington, Pa.: Eastern National, 2000), 167.
6. Dan McNichol, *The Roads That Built America* (New York: Sterling, 2006), chapter 6.

CHAPTER 2: DIFFERENT MODELS, COMMON PRINCIPLES

1. WHO, *The World Health Report, 2000,* Annex Table 8, p. 195.
2. See, e.g., Eric Noe, "Toyota, Honda Gaining on U.S. Automakers," ABC News, November 22, 2005, http://abcnews.go.com/Business.
3. Author interview with Tsung-Mei Cheng, November 10, 2007.

CHAPTER 3: THE PARADOX

1. The Commonwealth Fund's National Scorecard reports provide careful and insightful comparative measures of national health systems. They are available at www. commonwealthfund.org and are regularly noted in the invaluable journal *Health Affairs.* See Cathy Schoen et al., "U.S. Health System Performance: A National Scorecard," *Health Affairs* Web Exclusive, September 20, 2006, p. W457.
2. WHO, *The World Health Report, 2000,* Annex Table 7, p. 189.
3. David Himmelstein et al., "MarketWatch: Illness and Injury As Contributors to Bankruptcy," *Health Affairs* Web Exclusive, February 2, 2005, pp. W5-62.
4. Ellen Nolte et al., "Measuring the Health of Nations: Updating an Earlier Analysis," *Health Affairs,* January/February 2008, p. 71.
5. The Commonwealth Fund, *Multinational Comparisons of Health Systems Data,* November 2006.
6. Schoen et al., "U.S. Health System Performance."
7. Ibid.
8. Patricia Danzon, "Liability for Medical Malpractice," *Handbook of Health Economics,* vol. 1B (Burlington, Ma.: Elsevier, 2000), chapter 26.
9. Jim Landers, "Malpractice Damage Caps Not a Cure for High Health Care Costs," *Dallas Morning News,* May 5, 2010.
10. For example, see "UnitedHealth Slashes Forecast," *Wall Street Journal,* April 23, 2008, p. B4; PULSE (newsletter), September 2005, p. 1.
11. An ace reporter, Lisa Girion of the *Los Angeles Times,* has reported in depth on the industry's selection practices. See, e.g., Lisa Girion, "Insurers Reject Applications of Some Individuals with Minor Ailments," *Los Angeles Times,* December 31, 2006.
12. Vanessa Furhmans, "Fights Over Health Claims," *Wall Street Journal,* February 14, 2007, p. A1.

13. European Observatory on Health Systems and Policies, *Funding Health Care: Options for Europe*, 2002.

14. Henry Aaron, "The Costs of Health Care Administration in the U.S. and Canada," *New England Journal of Medicine*, August 21, 2003, p. 801.

CHAPTER 4: FRANCE: THE VITAL CARD

1. Dr. Péan's innovation is described in Richard J. Friedman, ed., *Arthroplasty of the Shoulder* (New York: Thieme, 1994), 1–2.

2. The Commonwealth Fund, *Multinational Comparisons of Health Systems Data*, November 2006.

3. WHO, *The World Health Report, 2000*, Annex Table 4.

4. For an excellent description of the French system, see Victor G. Rodwin et al., *Universal Health Insurance in France—How Sustainable?* (Washington, D.C.: Embassy of France, 2006). Much of the statistical information here comes from the Rodwin volume.

5. Kerry Capell, "The French Lesson in Health Care," *BusinessWeek*, July 9, 2007.

6. *Wall Street Journal*, January 25, 2007, p. C1.

7. Rodwin et al., *Universal Health Insurance in France*, p. 31.

8. Ibid., p. 67.

9. Rodwin et al., *Universal Health Insurance in France*, pp. 10–11.

CHAPTER 5: GERMANY: "APPLIED CHRISTIANITY"

1. "Waiting Times for Care?" *Medical News Today*, July 10, 2007.

2. Katherine Anne Lehrman, *Bismarck: Profiles in Power* (London: Pearson, 2004), 6. Another excellent source on Bismarck, his life, and his welfare state innovations is Edgar Feuchtwanger, *Bismarck* (Milton Park, UK: Routledge, 2002).

3. Laurene Gregg, *The Health of Nations* (Congressional Quarterly Books, 1999), 49.

4. Speeches of Otto von Bismarck, Bavarian State Library, Münchener Digitalisierungszentrum (MDZ), p. 165.

5. Werner Richter, *Bismarck* (New York: G.P. Putnam's Sons, 1965), 275.

CHAPTER 6: JAPAN: BISMARCK ON RICE

1. The usage statistics were compiled by Ikegami Naoki. See Ikegami, *Iryou Mondai* (Nihon Keizai Shimbun Shuppansha, 2007) (in Japanese).
2. J. C. Campbell and N. Ikegami, *The Art of Balance in Health Policy* (Cambridge: Cambridge University Press, 1998), 53–86.

CHAPTER 7: THE UK: UNIVERSAL COVERAGE, NO BILLS

1. An excellent study of William Beveridge's eventful life, and the main source I used, is Jose Harris, *William Beveridge: A Biography* (Oxford: Oxford University Press, 1977).
2. Harris, *William Beveridge*, p. 390.
3. Among several good biographies of Bevan, I relied primarily on John Campbell, *Aneurin Bevan and the Mirage of British Socialism* (New York: W. W. Norton, 1987).
4. In the House of Commons, December 6, 1945 (Hansard, vol. 411).
5. Eric Shaw, *The Labour Party since 1945* (Blackwell, 1996), 39.
6. Thomas Bodenheimer and Kevin Grumbach, *Understanding Health Policy: A Clinical Approach* (Lange Medical Books, 2005), 151.
7. Ibid.

CHAPTER 8: CANADA: "SORRY TO KEEP YOU WAITING"

1. Walter Stewart, *The Life and Times of Tommy Douglas* (McArthur, 2003), chapter 2.
2. T. C. Douglas, *The Making of a Socialist* (Edmonton: McClelland & Stewart, 1975), 17.
3. Laurie J. Goldsmith, *Canada,* in EU Observer, The Wealthy Countries, 2000, p. 227.
4. Steven Katz et al., "Phantoms in the Snow: Canadians' Use of Health Care Services in the U.S.," *Health Affairs,* May/June 2002, p. 19.
5. Douglas, *The Making of a Socialist*, p. 59.
6. Author interview with Noel Doig,
7. From the CBC Web site: "In November 2004, Canadians voted Tommy

Douglas the Greatest Canadian of all time following a nationwide contest. Over 1.2 million votes were cast in a frenzy of voting that took place over six weeks." To read more, go to http://www.cbc.ca/greatest/.

8.   *British Medical Journal,* June 18, 2005, p. 1408. The full text of the Supreme Court opinion can be found at http://www.canlii.org/en/ca/scc/doc/2005 /2005scc35/2005scc35.html.

CHAPTER 9: OUT OF POCKET

1.   Thomas P. Ofcansky et al., *Ethiopia: A Country Study* (Washington, D.C.: Government Printing Office, 1991), "Health and Welfare," p. 1.

2.   WHO, *World Medicines Strategy, 2001,* http://ftp.who.int/gb/archive/pdf_files/WHA54/ea54r11.pdf.

3.   American Enterprise Institute, *Medicinal Malpractice: Improving Drug Access,* Health Policy Outlook No. 10, December 2006.

4.   "Uninsured Adults More Likely to Die Prematurely," press release, National Academy of Sciences, May 21, 2002.

5.   WHO, *The World Health Report, 2004,* Annex Table 1, p. 112.

6.   D. Blumenthal and W. Hsiao, "Privatization and Its Discontents," *New England Journal of Medicine,* September 15, 2005, p. 1168.

7.   Ibid.

8.   You can read about these and other exotic therapies on the NCCAM Web site, http://nccam.nih.gov/.

CHAPTER 10: TOO BIG TO CHANGE?

1.   Ezra Klein, "The Lessons of '94," *The American Prospect,* January 22, 2008 (Web only).

2.   Reinhard Busse et al., *Health Care Systems in Transition* (Germany: European Observatory on Health Systems and Policies, 2004).

3.   Author interviews with William Hsiao and Chang Hong-Jen, October 22, 2007.

4.   Tsung-Mei Cheng, "Taiwan's New National Health Insurance Program," *Health Affairs,* May/June 2003.

5.   CIA, *The World Factbook,* 2010.

6. Author interview with Swiss health minister Ruth Dreyfus, October 29, 2007.

7. The best study of the Clinton health care plan was the work of two reporters who were my mentors at the *Washington Post*. See Haynes Johnson and David Broder, *The System: The American Way of Politics at the Breaking Point* (Boston: Little, Brown & Co., 1996).

CHAPTER 11: AN APPLE A DAY

1. Ian Urbina, "In the Treatment of Diabetes," *New York Times*, January 11, 2006, p. 1.

2. Ibid.

3. *CAA Cancer Journal for Clinicians* 4 (1954): 47–48. Available online at http://caonline.amcancersoc.org/cgi/reprint/4/2/470.

4. Quoted in *The Oxford Handbook of Public Health Practice* (Burlington, Ma.: Elsevier, 2002).

5. All the data on health inequalities due to income come from Thomas Bodenheimer and Kevin Grumbach, *Understanding Health Policy: A Clinical Approach* (Large Medical Books, 2005), 25.

6. Ibid., p. 109.

7. Charles F. Mullett, *The Bubonic Plague and England* (Lexington: University of Kentucky Press, 1956), chapter 2.

8. From the author's collection of international cigarette pack warnings.

9. Joshua T. Cohen et al., "Does Preventive Care Save Money?" *New England Journal of Medicine,* February 14, 2008.

CHAPTER 12: THE FIRST QUESTION

1. Institute of Medicine, *Care Without Coverage: Too Little, Too Late* (2002).

2. Urban Institute, *Uninsured and Dying Because of It: Updating the Institute of Medicine Analysis on the Impact of Uninsurance on Mortality* (2008). Available online at www.urban.org/Uploaded PDF/411588_uninsured_dying .pdf.

3. Andrew P. Wilper et al., "Health Insurance and Mortality in US Adults," *American Journal of Public Health* 99, no. 12 (December 2009): 2289–2295.

4. "Treatments," Lupus Foundation Web site, www.lupus.org.

5. Article 25. Full text of the universal declaration is available at www.un.org/Overview/rights.html.

6. Article 12. Full text of the international covenant is available at www.unhchr.ch/html/menu3/b/a_cescr.htm.

7. André Den Exter et al., *The Right to Health Care in Several European Countries* (Alphen aan den Rijn, Netherlands: Kluwer 1995), 40.

8. Article 35. Full text of the charter is available online at http://www.europarl.europa.eu/charter/default_en.htm.

9. Den Exter et al., *The Right to Health Care*, p. 156.

10. On KING-TV, March 13, 2007.

11. George W. Bush, Town Meeting, Cleveland, Ohio, July 10, 2007, at www.whitehouse.gov/briefing_room.

12. Scott Becker, *Health Care Law: A Practical Guide*, 2008, Sec. 21.01(3).

13. William J. Clinton, State of the Union address, February 17, 1993.

14. "Wanted: A Clearly Articulated Social Ethic for American Health Care," *JAMA,* November 5, 1997, p. 1447.

15. "Letters," *JAMA,* March 11, 1998.

AN AFTERWORD: "OBAMACARE"

1. Congressional Budget Office, "Cost Estimates for Health Care Legislation," http://www.cbo.gov/publications/collections/health.cfm.

2. For a good description of the two prongs, see Kaiser Family Foundation, "Focus on Health Reform," 4/21/10, http://www.kff.org/healthreform/upload/8061.pdf.

3. Congressional Budget Office, "Cost Estimates for Health Care Legislation," http://www.cbo.gov/publications/collections/health.cfm.

APPENDIX: THE BEST HEALTH CARE SYSTEM IN THE WORLD

1. CIA, The World Factbook, at https://www.cia.gov/library/publications/the-world-factbook/.

2. Thomas Bodenheimer and Kevin Grumbach, *Understanding Health Policy: A Clinical Approach* (Large Medical Books, 2005), p. 109.

3. The DALE concept is explained in WHO, *The World Health Report, 2000,* pp. 27–29.

4. Ceri Phillips and Guy Thompson, "What Is a QALY?," Hayward Medical Communications (2001), pp. 1–6.

5. Ibid.

6. WHO, *The World Health Report, 2000,* p. vii.

7. Robert Blendon et al., "The Public Versus the World Health Organization," *Health Affairs,* May/June 2001, p. 16.

8. Cathy Schoen et al., *Health Affairs* Web Exclusive, November/December 2006, p. W457.

9. Heritage Foundation, *Backgrounder No. 1973,* September 22, 2006.

Index